AF605906

EMBODIED NARRATIVES IN THE HEALTH HUMANITIES AND LITERARY STUDIES

# Embodied Narratives in the Health Humanities and Literary Studies

EDITED BY EFTIHIA MIHELAKIS AND LUCILLE TOTH

UNIVERSITY OF TORONTO PRESS
Toronto Buffalo London

Toronto Buffalo London
utppublishing.com
Printed in Canada

ISBN 978-1-4875-5942-7 (cloth) ISBN 978-1-4875-5944-1 (EPUB)
ISBN 978-1-4875-5943-4 (PDF)

**Library and Archives Canada Cataloguing in Publication**

Title: Embodied narratives in the health humanities and literary studies / edited by Eftihia Mihelakis and Lucille Toth.
Names: Mihelakis, Eftihia, 1982– editor | Toth, Lucille, editor
Description: Includes bibliographical references and index.
Identifiers: Canadiana (print) 20250289024 | Canadiana (ebook) 20250289105 | ISBN 9781487559427 (cloth) | ISBN 9781487559434 (PDF) | ISBN 9781487559441 (EPUB)
Subjects: LCSH: Narrative medicine. | LCSH: Literature and medicine.
Classification: LCC RC48 .E43 2025 | DDC 610.69/6—dc23

Cover design: Val Cooke

Cover image: Darian Goldin Stahl, "Glory," Ink transfer, 30" x 22," 2021. Image courtesy of the artist. To see more of Stahl's work, please visit her website, www.dariangoldinstahl.com

We wish to acknowledge the land on which the University of Toronto Press operates. This land is the traditional territory of the Wendat, the Anishnaabeg, the Haudenosaunee, the Métis, and the Mississaugas of the Credit First Nation.

This book has been published with the help of a grant from the Federation for the Humanities and Social Sciences, through the Awards to Scholarly Publications Program, using funds provided by the Social Sciences and Humanities Research Council of Canada.

University of Toronto Press acknowledges the financial support of the Government of Canada, the Canada Council for the Arts, and the Ontario Arts Council, an agency of the Government of Ontario, for its publishing activities.

Canada Council for the Arts Conseil des Arts du Canada

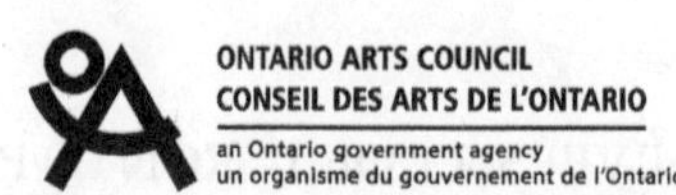


Funded by the Government of Canada | Financé par le gouvernement du Canada | Canada

# Contents

# Acknowledgements

We extend our deepest gratitude to the authors of the chapters whose contributions shaped this volume and the fields of literary studies and health humanities in a meaningful way.

We thank our editor Jodi Litvin for her dedicated and enthusiastic support throughout the process of writing this book and Natalie Garriga for her attention to detail throughout the revisions and proofs.

Our recognition also goes out to the reviewers whose thorough and thoughtful observations opened up key considerations around the ways in which health care cannot be reduced to its biomedical aspects. Their recognition of how the arts shape this field through the ways in which they rethink, remap, reshape, and trouble health gave us hope to pursue the book by paying special attention to the significance of the embodiment of care. As such, we want to make sure their insight is recognized here. We acknowledge with heartfelt appreciation the ways in which the book emerges, travels, and positively rethinks patient agency and narrative conventions of illness.

We also want to express our deepest gratitude to Dr. Darian Goldin Stahl for her evocative cover illustration that visually captures the spirit of this book, lending it a distinctive and compelling aesthetic that we feel not only enhances the text, but also resonates with the ways in which art is embedded within, and helps to shape, a broader network of discourses around health equity.

This book would not have been possible without the financial support of the Awards to Scholarly Publications Program, the Department of French and Italian of the Ohio State University-Newark, and the Social Sciences and Humanities Research Council, through the Insight Development Grant in Research-Creation awarded to Dr. Eftihia Mihelakis for her project *Ce qui gît sous la pourssière: Écritures de la depression en contextes de marginalisations* (# 430-2022-00525).

EMBODIED NARRATIVES IN THE HEALTH HUMANITIES AND LITERARY STUDIES

# Embodying Narratives in the Health Humanities and Literary Studies: An Introduction

EFTIHIA MIHELAKIS AND LUCILLE TOTH

Le sens du mot, n'est pas contenu dans le mot comme son. Mais c'est la définition du corps humain de s'approprier dans une série indéfinie d'actes discontinus des noyaux significatifs qui dépassent et transfigurent ses pouvoirs naturels.

– Merleau-Ponty, *Phénoménologie de la perception*

The patient's place in society, in his or her family, must be maintained. This is why the patient has to have a social attitude: writing, receiving news and narrating are some of the most important social activities.

– Fanon, *Alienation and Freedom*

The literary productions examined in this book share the conviction that the act of writing is physically demanding. Drawing from Maurice Merleau-Ponty's account of the *Erlebnis*, "lived experience" is both lived and corporeal. It transcends passivity for it is the very means through which we engage with and comprehend our surroundings. Working as "acts of consciousness" (466), the texts presented in this volume embody strategies developed in the Global North and the Global South and endorse the significance of material phenomenology. This perspective resonates deeply with the work of anti-colonial psychiatrist Frantz Fanon, who recognized the radical and therapeutic potential of first-person narratives in addressing the psychosomatic repercussions of colonial and racial oppression. Fanon's establishment of the weekly psychiatric unit newspaper *Notre Journal* at the Hôpital Blida-Joinville in colonial Algeria in 1953 provided a refuge for patients, staff, and doctors to contribute and write as a form of *narrative repair*. Fanon "consecrated the therapeutic importance of reclaiming language, which was denied to [his] patients due to mental illness, but also [through forms] of alienation, dispossession, and silencing inflicted [on them] by colonization" (Beckman et al. 180). His insights, articulated in both *Black Skin, White Masks* (1952) and *A Dying Colonialism* (1959), reveal how psychological distress can manifest as physical symptoms, offering tangible strategies to address somatic ailments stemming from the trauma of colonial violence and racial discrimination, such as anxiety, depression, and other psychosomatic illnesses. Predating the formal establishment of embodied cognition as a theoretical framework, Merleau-Ponty's and Fanon's perspectives of the embodied experience of oppression and perception align closely with the core tenets of our own understanding of embodiment.

In the last thirty years, *embodiment* has occupied a central place in cognitive science and human experience. Here, we take Varela et al.'s *The Embodied Mind* (1991) as a work that pioneers the field. *The Embodied Mind* introduces the concept of "enaction," which emphasizes the active role the body plays in its environment, shaping cognition and consciousness. Since then, embodiment has become a key term through which to consider health and illness as valuable epistemic tools, a way of framing our (mis)understandings of the relationship between the way our bodies speak and the way we attempt to tell their stories. While language is commonly recognized as *dis*embodied, claiming that language is intricately connected to our bodily encounters crucially empowers embodiment theory as more than just a disincarnated epistemic framework.

We recognize that the "we" we display in this introduction is typographically, physically, and socially enacted. Our subject positions embody our situated knowledge, which we experience through our bodies, and this is the main reason we have engaged with health humanities from both theoretical and research-creation perspectives. When we discuss our individual experiences here, we will use our initials (EM and LT). EM: I first began incorporating research-creation (then existing as an experience of binary tension) two decades ago, when as a French literature undergraduate student at McGill University, I found my emerging critical voice divided into two distinctly constructed arenas: either in theoretical courses or in creative writing courses. I had many excellent professors there, all attuned to the complex dimensions of each field, approach, and praxis. But my institutional philosophies and practices carried with them orientations that were originally designed (albeit not always directly or consciously) to divide the mind from the body, reifying the Western binary in which the intellect is housed in cerebral dimensions and creative writing in our mortal flesh. I craved a form (not yet named in the institution but starting to take form at the Université du Québec à Montréal where

I then went on to pursue a master's degree in literary studies) that would provide me with the space and the possibility to experiment and experience the unfolding of literary language through a research-led and arts-driven way. Since then, I have drawn on gender, sexuality, diasporic, and critical race studies that exceed linguistic and identity categories, as well as disciplinary bounds, revealing how liminal spaces are woven into thinking-artistic-spaces, those that are more than disciplinary (McCormack 1) and yet confined within the oft-contentious and complex boundaries of the academe. While research-creation has now become integral to my identity as both scholar and writer, I cannot overstate the need to engage with literary studies as an integral part of conducting academic projects in the health humanities. This thinking is deeply embedded in a translingual practice of reading, writing, and thinking that resists the "outsourcing" or disembodiment of literary knowledge processes towards more "useful" sciences (where works of literature are used or perceived as a set of texts, concepts, or tools to fit an already-chosen orientation), or "less risky" epistemic positionalities, or more "popular/accessible" languages (i.e., English).

As a dance and medical humanities scholar, I (LT) investigate how dance functions as a unique grammar for expressing the struggles and challenges faced by marginalized groups, particularly within the contexts of pandemics and migration. My exploration of the medical humanities began by examining the repercussions of the HIV/AIDS pandemic on dancers, while also questioning the medical and esthetic ramifications of the sexual exploitation of nineteenth-century dancers in France. As a creative-research scholar, I collaborated with photographers and choreographers to examine topics such as intimacy in the post-AIDS era and cultural myths surrounding women and hysteria. Through these collaborations and my own practice as a mover, I re-evaluate the place of viral narratives in the COVID-19 era and reassess the ways in which pandemics compel researchers and practitioners towards intellectual creativity and activism. At a time when environmental and health crises are impossible to disconnect, together, we contend that we require wild, complex, even opaque ways of sharing our human, not-so-human, and planetary health.

This is the reason we have collaborated with the fourteen authors present in this book: here, fat studies, queer studies, gender studies, critical race studies, and dance studies, as well as research-creation, cohabitate with health humanities and literary studies to provide a working impulse of the present-day bio-politics, aesthetics, and ethics in the cultures in which literary studies do not contend only with the rise of health humanities.

Together, we look at the tensions and challenges that arise through literary studies, particularly whether these narrative structures are patient- and/or artist-activist-led instead of asking whether literary studies *can* change the world, that is, whether it has the power to move the world. While we understand that we cannot overcome or ignore the politically inflected demands and tensions that have marked and that continually mark our world, we have consciously and conscientiously chosen to move away from methods of deconstructing or unmasking the incapacities of the literary to overcome suffering, marginalization, violence, and injustice to focus at *how* the literary produces different types of attachments through its own language, *through* the potential of textuality as embodiment. If we question neo-liberalistic and silence-generating imperatives surrounding individualistic sociocultural systems that have failed to afford a measure of inherent worth, we do so in ways that aim to provide access and attention to the literary impetus in the realm of auto/biographical and narrative studies.

## Embodying (Our) Academic Strategies

*Embodied Narratives in the Health Humanities and Literary Studies* offers a critical and creative framework for understanding the move towards embodied narratives of health, ones that are attuned to exploring the shift in power that can take place in long-standing discourses regarding the experience of disease and illness, whether literary, cultural, or historical. Embodied narratives of health have the potential to "leave room for creative spaces: unfinished sites that represent the possibilities" (Sarr 109) of health humanities. The concern of addressing (How do we address?) embodied narratives in health humanities and literary studies is in no way a univocal issue, and we contend that it is not limited to narrative medicine. Until recently, literary studies – understood in its transnational sense for transdisciplinary reflection on personal and social discourses pertaining to health, medicine, nursing, and the diverse implications of health humanities – had received limited scholarly attention. However, a growing body of work, including Jennifer Boum Make's *Decolonial Care* (2025) and Elsner and Pietrzak-Franger's edited volume *Literature and Medicine* (2024), signals a renewed interest in the field. Our volume aligns with this emerging scholarship, contributing tools for analyzing literary forms that explore the medicalized body and its impact on contemporary life beyond clinical practice. There is a significant lack of scholarly tools that allow for the analysis and assessment of the undeniably growing production and popularity of literary forms focusing on the fate of the medicalized body and its impact on contemporary living, but that are not meant to serve the clinical practice a priori. In this book, these configurations are creating new experiences of cohabitation, real or imagined, across geographies and within the fabric of societies.

As health humanities scholars working through the literary studies, our positionality is impacted by the COVID-19 pandemic and the way it challenged the field of health humanities. Our choice to focus on work within and through the *health* humanities as opposed to the *medical* humanities is rooted in the belief that social and cultural determinants of health, health policy, and disparities influence health and healthcare. By offering a holistic approach which allows stronger emphasis on social justice, health equity, and advocacy, health humanities offer community-based projects with practical applications of patient advocacy efforts. We hope that this book opens the discussion around current debates and discourses, most notably, regarding the institutional relevance of knowledge production and hierarchical power dynamics concerning ownership of what constitutes valid or valuable knowledge for the transdisciplinary field. While many humanities and social sciences scholars are contending and engaging with the growing prominence of research-creation across Canada (Loveless; Mavrikakis; Martelly; Truman), and specifically around the connections between research-creation and the health humanities (Goldin Stahl; Gendron et al.; Mavrikakis et al.; Neilson et al.; Peacock and Peterson) as a way to question and re-evaluate the relationship between arts practices, theory, and research (Truman and Springhay), an array of stories and bodies are resonating with one another in complex ways that challenge our neo-liberal impetus to find fast and rapid solutions that can remedy our issues. The literary demands that we understand the health humanities as encompassing a spectrum of narrative practices that, in turn, allow us to consider the limits and possibilities of embodied narratives and somatic experiences.

Historically, the perspective of the medical humanities gained momentum at the end of the twentieth century and the beginning of the twenty-first century as part of the wider need within (Western) medical education programs to "extend empathy toward those who suffer, and to join honestly and courageously with patients in their struggles toward recovery, with chronic illness, or in facing death" (Charon 3). There was also a pedagogical and training imperative to enhance attention on narrative medicine as a way to bridge the gap between evidence-based care and medical humanities (Marini). Narrative medicine as a study was introduced by general internist and literary scholar Rita Charon in 2001. Its central focus is "the clinical applications of literary knowledge"

(Charon et al.). It explores what literature can do in the field of medicine by being "attentive to the relational dynamics at work in every human encounter" (Charon et al. 18). Narrative medicine therefore attempts to use the method of analyzing literary works for patient-to-doctor interviews in a medical field and tries to cultivate narrative competency and relationality through the practice of close reading and writing as therapy. As Craig Irvine and Rita Charon asserted in their chapter "Deliver Us from Certainty: Training for Narrative Ethics," "Narrative practices are not only the therapeutic means, but the therapy itself" (vi), not subordinate to medical care but the essence of medical care. Narrative medicine has been steadily growing, with medical humanities programs and departments multiplying across Canada and the United States, and it has been developed as a medical education tool (Milota et al.) with the aim to create more empathetic medical practitioners.

The influential discipline of narrative medicine, in the words of Rita Charon at the time of its establishment, made no secret that the nature of its practice was clinical. Furthermore, it defined its goal as a practice of medicine "with ... the narrative skills of recognizing, absorbing, interpreting, and being moved by the stories of illness," the assumption behind such a skill-set acquisition being that "the reader of a novel or the witness of a drama ... naturally do all these things seamlessly" (Charon 4). Literary studies scholars, artist-scholars, and/or health humanities artists and/or scholars working tangentially with/in the literary studies would surely respond differently to such an approach, most notably that of questioning the viability of making adjunct the literary to the medical, or even agreeing with the postulate that literature and embodied narratives can actually be useful for medical care. Accordingly, our volume aligns itself with the more recent work produced by Anna M. Elsner and Monika Pietrzak-Franger that openly "scrutinize[s] discourses of use," contending that even when literature can exist in a reciprocal relationship with medicine (and its institution), because it produces "divergence, difference, and complexity," we must resist the urge of instrumentalism for the sake of building certain skills in doctors and/or tools for patients. If the potential of literature to represent "medical practice, healthcare, physicians, nurses, patients, and family members caring for the ill span all historical periods and transcend languages and cultures" has existed since time immemorial, we seek to emphasize the relationship between two fields (one with a history stemming from the nineteenth century, literary studies, and the other surfacing from the need to include and examine the intricate relationship between health and the human condition, health humanities).

Recent studies within the field of health humanities and embodiment, as evidenced by the works of Boileau and Johnson, as well as DeTora and Cressman, rely on the combination between text and image. Notably, DeTora and Cressman's work showcases the profound role of graphic novels as it relates to the ways in which it can help those who experience illness as well as their caregivers to "enhance their ability ... to share their stories" (DeTora and Cressman 15). Artist and scholar Darian Goldin Stahl's *Embodied Books* project exemplifies innovative and therapeutic practices that employ both text and imagery to explore the embodied dimensions of illness and healthcare. Using the materiality and plasticity of books, participants engage in crafting artists' books centred on their personal experiences with healthcare. Similarly, dance/movement therapy (DMT) offers a distinct avenue to embodied narratives of health, or kinesthetic narratives, wherein the body communicates stories through its movements. "Conscious body movements generate a fluid, nonverbal narration of self and identity no less important than the verbal stories we may tell" (Caldwell 89).

For us, the impetus of embodiments represents an ongoing process that exists at the crossroad at which narratives collide with the health humanities. This collision serves as a fertile site, a space for imagining real and fictional (and everything in between) forms of embodiment thus highlighting the im/possibilities of a convergence between text, image, body, and culture. The literary productions delving into the medicalized body and its implications for our contemporary world bear witness to a burgeoning interest in narratives of illness. These manifestations are made possible when close reading; medical, ethical, and legal critical theory; feminist and intersectional analysis; self-reflective narratives; neurolinguistics; cultural history; reparative forms of critique; and aesthetics collide. We aim to lay the groundwork for future transdisciplinary research, teaching endeavours, and artistic pursuits.

## Consolidating Translingual and Transdisciplinary Frameworks

In this book, we are committed to a transdisciplinary imaginative endeavour of literary studies. Although there is still no clear consensus on this specific endeavour's ontological architecture, we have found energy in the still nascent but rapidly growing conversations around the need "to solve real-world problems that are complex, multidimensional and not confined by boundaries of a single disciplinary framework" (Wickson et al. 1046). Our aspiration with this book is to expand and chart new pathways for literary studies. This aspiration is evidenced partly by the surge in critical theory since the 1970s and the field's transnational turn (Jay). We pay heed to the complexities of borders concerning identities – be they national, regional, or personal. This shift in literary studies entails a departure from Eurocentric dominance, encouraging an examination of literature through an intersectional lens. We aim to illuminate how texts navigate and reflect upon the intricate intersections of identity and power dynamics. While our focus may not explicitly delve into the topic of globalization as it pertains to health humanities and literary studies, our objective remains attuned to one of its consequential by-products: language and hegemony. Indeed, we often attribute success to language's ability to reach a broad audience. However, our investigation into the embodiment of illness or health necessitates scrutiny of our capacity – or lack thereof – to "cohere" (Ahmed, *Queer Phenomenology* 170) within any one autonomous state of being.

Here, we engage with the notion of transnationalism by questioning the extensions and connections of the body's borders. Taking Vandebosch and D'haen's position as one significant starting point for our book, we look to engage with the transnational turn in literary studies by connecting with what "takes place in the liminal spaces between real and imagined borders" (Jay 1). Though we do not directly address national borders or the migration of individuals between nation states, our examination looks into the dynamics between marginalized and dominant groups. We also examine the evolving concerns surrounding categories, methodologies, and tools in an era marked by the coexistence of multiple identities. These identities are intricately linked to – or sometimes detached from – the epistemologies and methodologies concerning health, illness, and/or disability. Where this book lacks in its ability to "cohere" (Ahmed, *Queer Phenomenology* 170) to a narrative medicine viewpoint it gains in its willingness to pursue some possibilities that open the space for looking at the tensions that arise between "the perpetuation of domination based on class, gender, and race" (Vergès 3–4), the "normative ideas of health and ability" (Van Dam, this volume), where "queer moments" (Gagnon Chainey, this volume) not only articulate the desire to differentiate but ascertain the relationship between "colonial knowledge" (Kim, this volume), instrumentalist methods of scientific research (Raymond Bock, this volume), and state policing and discourses (Gilman, this volume).

The endeavour within narrative medicine to acknowledge the significance of embodied knowledge finds its roots in substantial shifts in scholarly priorities and analytical methodologies from the latter half of the twentieth century into the twenty-first century. These shifts have compelled scholars to scrutinize literature through ethical lenses, contemplating its moral implications and its potential for engaging with social justice issues. Notably, anglophone and francophone perspectives in literary studies exhibit divergent theoretical frameworks, critical approaches, and emphases. While both traditions grapple with ethical concerns, anglophone literary studies lean heavily towards postcolonial theory, feminist theory, queer theory, and critical race theory, while francophone literary studies are more influenced by post-structuralism, psychoanalysis, and semiotics. As scholars move away from the concept of "art for art's sake" towards exploring embodied theories (crip theory, among others), they are increasingly examining the ethical aspects inherent in literary texts. This movement also encompasses literary activism and advocacy within the discipline, aligning with the transdisciplinary approach of health humanities, which aims to comprehend medicine within its broader social, cultural, and ethical contexts. This involves addressing issues such as representation, power dynamics, and the responsibilities of authors; contesting prevailing narratives; and amplifying the voices of marginalized communities. These shifts in scholarly focus resonate with the principles of narrative medicine, which prioritize personal narratives, empathy, and ethical introspection within healthcare, but they do not necessarily comply with the objectives of narrative medicine.

The history of settler colonialism has decimated linguistic diversity as part of a larger design to magnify and elevate settler linguistic ideologies. Language affects every aspect of our life. Language is a vector of domination and oppression. Language can be slippery, ambiguous, clumsy, reassuring, empowering. With a simple set of spoken or written words, we can quicken someone's sense of comfort in their moment of distress just like we can ignite exclusion in ourselves or in others. What counts as a homologous, universally shared language, is integral to producing measures of whose bodies, whose lives, whose illness(es), whose suffering(s) dominate global knowledge production, research methods, and the affective and theoretical framing of a shared sense of belonging, caring (for), and speaking in the name of what and who counts.

While this book is written in English, we believe it can become a useful Trojan Horse. To quote French radical lesbian feminist Monique Wittig, language can operate like a "war machine" (75) upon the hegemonic context of anglocentrism when it attempts to unveil words as they are woven into theoretical and/or practice-based approaches that would be used in a familiar (i.e., anglophone) environment, but in the context of this book they have shifted orientation. Orientations "affect how we think ... . [They shape] ... how bodies are directed towards things." (Ahmed, "Orientations Matter" 234) It is this very proximity to words and worlds that would otherwise be elsewhere ignored or unaccounted that we hold as part of a larger endeavour to be in dialogue with an approach that seeks to connect starting points, pulling our attention in some directions and in some ways more than others (e.g., connecting literary studies with health humanities instead of repeating the agreed-on dominance of narrative medicine for the health humanities). What is so important about the different language communities and academic traditions combined in this book is how they challenge the solipsism and isolationism that can too often plague literary studies, especially when English has become the dominant language of exchange and debate, and where writing can draw on a relatively narrow, Anglo-Saxon-dominated literature.

The pressure to publish in English in both the literary studies and the health humanities brings to the foreground a linguistic dimension that is felt directly or indirectly in all of the chapters in this book, and it is one that considers the possibility of thinking transnationally about embodied narratives. This book, and our approach more generally, is a challenge to what easily confines the scholarly imagination of health humanities and the linguistic landscape – whether bound by identity, language, or nationality – that flows therein, and in turn, to whom can become an artist, a patient, a thinker working with physical bodies and/as bodies of work.

The reader of this book, we hope, will recognize its language(s), take them into their cognitive world, much like the Trojans took the Horse into their city, completely unaware that the language that is so familiar to them (through the English-language words like *care, illness, memory*, etc.) is altered from its accustomed place and use and has begun to spread out into unsuspected orientations. It is our position in this book that this is the work of translingualism. As Sarah Dowling suggests, this term "has gained currency in applied linguistics, in transnational and diasporic literary studies, and in composition and rhetoric because it describes the capacity of languages to interact, influence, and transform one another" (4–5). The term also "highlights the ways in which English is understood as the most natural and appropriate way to" (3) produce valuable knowledge capable of crossing borders or to engage with a community of scholars and practitioners in the health humanities in a universally accepted language. Our book attends to the translingual condition of health humanities, one that explores the embodiment of different ways of experiencing, experimenting, thinking, being, living, teaching, writing, dying, and criticizing the levels of truth, power, or attention afforded to each of these movable states as they relate directly or indirectly to one another.

### Choreographing Bodies of Work

In the construction of this work, we have chosen to depart from the usual linear, historical, or dialectical method of analysis. Instead, we have opted for a style akin to choreography, weaving our texts together as a choreographed script of bodies resonating with one another to highlight the dialogic nature of this volume. By intertwining our texts in this manner, our aim is to elicit not only intellectual involvement but also emotional and embodied resonance, encouraging readers to actively participate in the intricate web of ideas, a network of cells, flesh, blood, and bones yearning through narrative for social, emotional, political, and affective (dis)connection. Therefore, **Part I** models new perspectives on how to theorize embodied health and illness narratives. From a neuroscience perspective, **Fernanda Pérez-Gay Juárez and Louise Toutée**'s exploration of the cognitive neuroscience of fiction underscores the profound impact of narrative engagement on our brains and behaviour, highlighting the potential of fiction to foster empathy and social cognition. Their research shows how immersive storytelling activates neural pathways associated with understanding others' emotions and intentions, suggesting that fiction can be a powerful tool in enhancing social connections and promoting psychological well-being. A novelist and researcher, **Maxime Raymond Bock** explores the portraiture of French-Canadian voyageur Alexis Saint-Martin by Dr. William Beaumont, a nineteenth-century American surgeon celebrated as the "father of gastric physiology." Raymond Bock reveals both Saint-Martin's contributions to significant scientific advancements and his multifaceted identity within the sociohistorical context of his time. Literary scholar **Chang-Hee Kim** offers a poignant reflection on the experiences of post-World War II Japanese Americans in Okada's *No-No Boy*. Emphasizing the enduring impact of historical trauma and resilience, Kim critically interrogates the pervasive manifestations of racism, ableism, sexism, classism, socialism, and capitalism prevalent in the 1950s Western (North American) society. Together, these three texts delve into the nuanced exploration of historical narratives and lived experiences, presenting characters and figures as multifaceted individuals whose identities extend beyond sensationalized dimensions. This complexity mirrors the intricate neural pathways involved in processing narrative content, suggesting that our engagement with literature involves more than just cognitive processes – it encompasses a deep understanding of human experiences and perspectives.

**Part II** focuses on queer health narratives. American cultural and literary historian **Sander L. Gilman** shows that, in the context of the

COVID-19 pandemic, the virus occupies a paradoxical position of ubiquity and elusiveness, concurrently perceived as omnipresent yet also questioned in its existence, often attributed to various conspiracy theories. Gilman's exploration of the COVID-19 pandemic illuminates the complex interplay between fear, rationality, and societal perceptions, offering critical insights into the challenges of public health communication. Throughout the scholarly examination undertaken in his chapter, French Canadian literary scholar **Benjamin Gagnon Chainey** elucidates the varied ways in which symptoms defy the symbolic rationale of normative corporealities, which adhere to a linear temporal paradigm. Drawing on Halberstam's formulation in *The Queer Art of Failure*, this analysis deviates from convention by embracing the queer, sombre, and temporally dislocated aesthetics portrayed in the works of Huysmans, Guibert, and Wojnarowicz. Theatre scholar and former finance officer with Doctors Without Borders **Eric Jorgensen** advocates the pedagogical virtue of teaching by disclosure. In the intimate essay he offers, Jorgensen investigates AIDS narratives in theatre, using the example of famous Broadway composer Michael Friedman to explore how disclosing personal and collective stories about AIDS can serve as a powerful educational tool, fostering empathy and understanding among audiences. By examining Friedman's work and life, Jorgensen highlights the importance of transparency and vulnerability in teaching and storytelling, demonstrating how sharing real-life experiences can break down stigma and promote a deeper connection to the subject matter. Together, these texts emphasis on storytelling as a means of grappling with collective experiences reinforces the idea that narratives serve as powerful tools for fostering empathy, understanding, and social change.

**Part III** offers practice-based examples of health narratives. Medical humanities and literary scholar **Julie C. Van Dam**'s chapter showcases the ways in which graffiti activism serves as the "trait d'union" between health and community. For Van Dam, the nexus between feminist activism and physical and mental well-being is symbiotic, with activists navigating multiple challenges, including the pressures of neo-liberalism. These artist-activists advocate for a decolonial conception of health and care deeply rooted in communal solidarity, embodying what Achille Mbembe terms as the "active will to community" – a manifestation of the fundamental drive for life (*Out of the Dark Night* 2–3). Van Dam's examination of graffiti activism underscores the transformative potential of street art as a tool for social change and community empowerment. **Aude Bandini and Jonathan Garfinkel**'s investigation of various perspectives (personal, phenomenological, moral, social, and political) on the DIYAPS movement, or do-it-yourself artificial pancreas systems, highlights the democratization of healthcare through patient empowerment, challenging traditional notions of doctor-patient dynamics. This movement not only empowers patients but also fosters a collaborative approach to healthcare, in which the expertise and experiences of patients are valued alongside those of medical professionals. Bandini and Garfinkel's work underscores the potential of DIYAPS to revolutionize chronic disease management, promoting greater autonomy, personalized care, and innovation driven by patient communities. **Darian Goldin Stahl**'s study of artists' books in medical education reveals the therapeutic potential of creative expression in illness narratives, fostering empathy and understanding among healthcare providers. By engaging with artists' books, Stahl proves that medical learners gain insight into the disparities experienced by patients, fostering a greater capacity for empathetic and accommodating care in their future practices. Furthermore, for the makers themselves, the meditative process of reflection and creation offered by crafting their book-bodies provides a space for creative flourishing and well-being amid the challenges of illness. Ultimately, the *Embodied Books* project highlights the potential for artists' books to facilitate meaningful reflections on illness experiences and contribute to more compassionate and patient-centred healthcare practices. **Hilary Offman**'s creative analysis of psychotherapeutic interactions offers valuable insights into the complexities of identity, shame, and empathy in therapeutic relationships. For Offman, the narrative of a psychotherapy journey offers a poignant illustration of how the intersecting identities of both therapist and patient intertwine in intricate ways, profoundly shaping the dynamics of patient care. Through an intersectional lens, it becomes evident that the shame associated with marginalized identities is deeply ingrained within our societal fabric, permeating every facet of our lives. Together, these chapters highlight the empowerment of individuals and communities in challenging traditional hierarchical structures, whether in healthcare provision or societal activism.

## WORKS CITED

Adorno, Theodor. *Aesthetic Theory*. Translated by Robert Hullot-Kentor, Continuum, 2002.

Ahmed, Sara. *Queer Phenomenology: Orientations, Objects, Others*. Duke UP, 2006.

–. "Orientations Matter." *New Materialisms: Ontology, Agency, and Politics*, edited by Diana Coole and Samantha Frost, Duke UP, 2010, pp. 234–57.

Beckman, Emily, Elizabeth Nelson, and Modupe Labode. "Voices from the Newspaper Club: Patient Life at a State Psychiatric Hospital (1988–1992)." *Journal of Medical Humanities*, vol. 43, no. 1, 2022, pp. 179–195. https://doi.org/10.1007/s10912-020-09617-7.

Boileau, Kendra, and Rich Johnson, editors. *COVID Chronicles: A Comics Anthology*. Graphic Mundi, 2021.

Boum, Make Jennifer. *Decolonial Care: Reimagining Caregiving in the French Caribbean*. Rutgers UP, 2025.

Caldwell, Christine. "Mindfulness and Bodyfulness: A New Paradigm." *Journal of Contemplative Inquiry*, vol. 1, 2014, pp. 77–96.

Charon, Rita. *Narrative Medicine: Honoring the Stories of Illness*. Oxford UP, 2006.

Charon, Rita, et al. *The Principles and Practice of Narrative Medicine*. Oxford UP, 2017.

DeTora, Lisa, and Jodi Cressman, editors. *Graphic Embodiments: Perspectives on Health and Embodiments in Graphic Narratives*. Leuven UP, 2021.

Dowling, Sarah, *Translingual Poetics: Writing Personhood Under Settler Colonialism*. U of Iowa P, 2018.

Eagleton, Terry. *The Ideology of the Aesthetic*. Wiley-Blackwell, 1991.

Elsner, Anna M., and Monika Pietrzak-Franger, editors. *Literature and Medicine*. Cambridge UP, 2024.

Fanon, Frantz. *A Dying Colonialism*. 1959. Grove Press, 1994.

–. *Black Skin, White Masks*. 1952. Grove Press, 2008.

–. *Alienation and Freedom*, edited and compiled by Jean Khalfa and Robert J. C. Young. Translated by Steven Corcoran, Bloomsbury Publishing, 2018.

Gendron, Karine, et al. *La réinvention organique dans les domaines de la culture et de la médecine*. Presses de l'Université Laval, 2024.

Goldin Stahl, Darian. *Embodied Books: Experiencing the Health Humanities Through Artists' Books*. Peter Lang, 2024.

Halberstam, Judith. *The Queer Art of Failure*. Duke UP, 2013.

Huysmans, Joris-Karl. *Against the Grain (À Rebours)*. Translated by Havelock Ellis, Dover Publications, 1969. *Internet Archive*, http://archive.org/details/againstgrainareb00huys.

Irvine, Craig, and Rita Charon. "Deliver Us from Certainty: Training for Narrative Ethics." *The Principles and Practice of Narrative Medicine*, edited by Rita Charon et al., Oxford UP, 2016, pp. 110–34.

Jay, Paul. *The Transnational Turn in Literary Studies*. Cornell UP, 2010.

Lestrade, Didier. *ACT UP. Une histoire*. Éditions Denoël, 2000.

Loveless, Nathalie, editor. *Knowing and Knots: Methodologies and Ecologies in Research-Creation*. U Alberta P, 2020.

Marini, Maria Giulia. *Narrative Medicine: Bridging the Gap between Evidence-Based Care and Medical Humanities*. Springer, 2016.

Martelly, Stéphane. *Le sujet opaque*. Éditions L'Harmattan, 2001.

Mavrikakis, Catherine. *Diamanda Galàs. Guerrière et Gorgone*. Héliotrope, 2014.
Mavrikakis, Catherine, et al. *Ça ne tourne pas rond*. Héliotrope, 2024.
Mbembe, Achille. *Out of the Dark Night: Essays on Decolonization*. Translated by Daniela Ginsburg, Columbia UP, 2021.
Merleau-Ponty, Maurice. *Phénomenologie de la perception*. Gallimard, 2005.
Mihelakis, Eftihia. *La virginité en question, ou les jeunes filles sans âge*. Presses de l'Université de Montréal, 2017.
Milota, Megan, et al. "Narrative Medicine as a Medical Education Tool: A Systemic Review." *Medical Teacher*, vol. 41, no. 7, 2019, pp. 802-810. https://doi.org/10.1080/0142159X.2019.1584274. Medline:30983460.
Neilson, Shane, et al., editors. *The COVID Journals. Health-Care Workers Write the Pandemic*. U of Alberta P, 2023.
Peacock, Margaret, and Erik L. Peterson. *A Deeper Sickness: Journal of America in the Pandemic Year*. Beacon Press, 2022.
Sarr, Felwine. *Afrotopia*. Translated by Drew Burke and Sarah Jones-Boardman, U of Minnesota P, 2019.
"Symptom (n.)." *Online Etymology Dictionary*, edited by Douglas Harper. https://www.etymonline.com/word/symptom. Accessed 1 Mar. 2025.
Toth, Lucille. *Danses et pandémies. Du sida à la covid-19*. Nota bene, 2023.
Truman, Sarah E. *Feminist Speculation and the Practice of Research-Creation: Writing Pedagogies and Intertextual Affects*. Routledge, 2022.
Truman, Sarah E., and Stephanie Springray. "The Primacy of Movement in Research-Creation: New Materialist Approaches to Art Research and Pedagogy." *Art's Teachings, Teaching's Art: Philosophical, Critical, and Educational Musings*, edited by Megan Laverty and Tyson Lewis, Springer, 2015, pp. 151–64.
Vandebosch, Dagmar, and Theo D'haen, editors. *Literary Transnationalism(s)*. Brill Rodopi, 2019.
Varela, Francisco, et al., editors. *The Embodied Mind: Cognitive Science and Human Experience*. MIT Press, 1991.
Vergès, Françoise. 2019. *A Decolonial Feminism*. Translated by Ashley J. Bohrer with the author, Pluto Press, 2021.
Wickson, Fern, et al. "Transdisciplinary Research: Characteristics, Quandaries and Quality." *Futures*, vol. 38, 2006, pp. 1046–59. http://doi.org/10.1016/j.futures.2006.02.011.
Wittig, Monique. *The Straight Mind and Other Essays*. Beacon Press, 1992.
Wojnarowicz, David. *Memories That Smell Like Gasoline*. Artspace, 1992.

# PART I

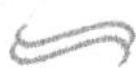

# Theorizing Embodied Health and Illness Narratives

# 1 The Cognitive Neuroscience of Literary Fiction: Bridging Biomedical Sciences and Health Humanities

FERNANDA PÉREZ-GAY JUÁREZ AND LOUISE TOUTÉE

Picture the following: A primate, from the family of the great apes, holds between its hands a squared object made of two plates of cardboard and multiple thin paper sheets in between, all tied together on one side. The great ape sits down, pulls the two cardboard plates – one with each hand – in a semi-circular motion, and the paper sheets reveal themselves. They are made of a whitish substance, with alternating patterns on top of similar-sized black marks that contrast with the white background, crossing it in horizontal lines. The great ape stares at the plates. If we look closely enough, we will notice how he starts moving his eyeballs, following these horizontal patterns of black marks, from left to right and then back to the right in the line below. This goes on for minutes, even hours. The ape uses his thumbs and index fingers to slide the paper sheets from right to left, one after another, once his eyes have reached the final line of black marks at the bottom of each one. At some point, he brings together the two cardboard plates, hiding the paper sheets again, and puts the object away.

From the observer's point of view, this was a repetitive set of behaviours happening in relative immobility. However, during this time, said great ape – which happens to be a human – traveled to a different time and place, experienced sequences of actions, visual scenes, social exchanges between recently met characters, and emotions. What exactly happened, at the biological level? This is, of course, an ambitious question to ask.

We know that those black marks on the pages have a name – words – and that they are the building blocks of language, a system of symbols that allows us to name, describe, and refer to instances in the world. We know that this language capability is one of the key features that differentiate humans from other species, including those primates closest to us from a genetic point of view. As biological organisms with a nervous system, the capacity to be somehow transported by staring at this object with words on it depends on the appropriate functioning of all our organs and systems, but one of these systems has a greater influence: the nervous system. Composed of the brain, the spinal cord, and the many nerves that go to our muscles and organs, our nervous system is organized in networks of interconnected neurons, cells that have the ability to send and receive electrochemical messages between them through junctions called *synapses*, transforming information from the outside world.

This biological set of synapses and neurons that reaches the most hidden corners in our body is the foundation on which the cultural inventions, including fictional universes, are built. In recent decades, the development of functional neuroimaging techniques, which allow measure brain activity to be measured while a subject performs a task, facilitated the fusion of neuroscience, which studies the biology of the nervous system, and cognitive psychology, which studies the functioning of the mind. This gave birth to cognitive neuroscience, which Nobel-Prize-winner Eric Kandel has referred to as "the new science of the mind" (546). When it comes to linguistics, functional brain imaging studies in cognitive neuroscience have revealed the location and time course of brain activity when deciphering written words, identifying the brain circuits through which we access their sounds and meanings (Dehaene). Furthermore, other studies have looked at the neurobiological activity that occurs during story comprehension (Mar) and narrative perception (Baldassano et al.), providing us with insights on the way our nervous systems treat the fictional situations we encounter in a book.

The purpose of the present article is to bring together these different aspects of cognitive neuroscience research that shed light on what happens in our nervous system when we engage with fictional narratives, from the way our visual systems process printed words in a book to the immersive experiences that can improve our understanding of ourselves, the world, and others, highlighting the potential for reading fiction to change our brains – and therefore our lives.

## The Linguistic Brain: From Words to Worlds

Linguistic functions were the first to be localized in the brain. The neurobiology of language was born in 1861, when French anthropologist and neurologist Pierre Paul Broca described a series of cases of patients who had lost the ability to emit coherent language, even if they could understand when spoken to and their vocal cords and articulatory phonetics were intact. In the post-mortem examination of these patient's brains, Broca found damage in the back of the left frontal lobe. This area, identified as the *seat of speech production*, was subsequently named after him, and the described clinical syndrome is today known as *Broca's aphasia* (Hickok et al.; Keller et al.).

Twelve years later, neurologist Karl Wernicke encountered patients with a different type of aphasia in his clinical practice. Although they articulated complete words, the subjects studied by Wernicke did not understand when spoken to and emitted sentences without logical sense. After studying their brains post-mortem, Wernicke found that the damaged area in these cases was in the upper part of the temporal lobe, in its junction with the parietal and occipital lobes. This area is today known as *Wernicke's area* and the type of comprehension aphasia he described is known as *Wernicke's aphasia* (Binder).

These lesion–symptom mapping discoveries set the groundwork to design the first neural model of language, which involved two separate systems that act in parallel: a sensory system of language – to perceive and understand it – located in the temporal lobe and a motor system – to produce and emit speech – in the frontal lobe, connected by the so-called arcuate fasciculus, a group of axons that go from one area to another, setting the basis for the brain circuitry of language production and understanding. This initial language model was refined by Geschwind, who tied it together with the brain's perception and movement systems and included the role of the right hemisphere in extracting and producing language tonality, or prosody.

In the last sixty years, the picture of the linguistic brain has grown increasingly complex. Modern neuroscience has shifted from the view that discrete brain regions are the seat of psychological function towards a network-based approach in which function derives not from a single area but from a set of interconnected regions that engage in *parallel processing*; that is, the initial sensory signals can travel through different routes at the same time and integrated in later stages (Bassett and Sporns). Nowadays, the model of the "core" language brain network considers two interacting pathways: one for language comprehension – organized bilaterally and lying in the temporal lobes – and one for language production – lateralized to the left, including Broca's area in the frontal lobe (Nasios et al.). This core network is mostly involved in formal linguistic functions, such as phonology, syntax and basic lexical functions. But to make these processes possible in the context of natural communication requires dynamic interaction with our physical and sociocultural environments (as we will see in the following sections); many other regions and networks are involved, including those relevant to action, perception, affect, social cognition and cognitive control, in what has been referred to as the extended language network (Hertrich et al.). This wide-spread activation of our neural circuits underlies our engagement with the literary arts. In the following sections, we will travel through the nervous paths that transform the words printed on a page to the worlds that narratives create in our mind.

## Reading in the Brain: Connecting Visual Input to Verbal Thought

Beyond the age-old debate about "nature versus nurture" in speech and language (Chomsky; Skinner), developmental studies have shown that human brains are prepared for oral language from birth. Infants exhibit universal patterns of speech perception and production before one year of age (Kuhl). During this time, they are especially good at hearing acoustic changes that differentiate phonemes even in languages they have never experienced (Eimas et al.), suggesting that the infant brain can crack the speech code in a way that the adult brain cannot.

Learning, of course, plays a fundamental role in oral language acquisition: To successfully develop linguistic capacities, this innate linguistic predisposition in infants has to be fed by social interaction with parents or caregivers throughout the first months of a baby's life, when they will learn to produce the phonemes of the language or languages they are exposed to by listening to and imitating adults (Kuhl and Meltzoff). Infants as young as three years old show activation in the same brain region responsible for speech production in adults – Broca's area – when hearing other people speak, showing that these early capabilities already depend on pre-established linguistic brain circuits (Dehaene-Lambertz et al.; Imada et al.).

In contrast to oral language, which has been hypothesized to have emerged at least 100,000 years ago (Lieberman), written language is a relatively recent acquisition, and we are not born with brain circuits ready to pick up on written words. However, after learning to read in school, we progressively develop the capacity to extract sounds and meanings quickly and accurately from written words (Dehaene). Research in the cognitive neuroscience of reading suggests that learning to read changes our brain circuitry: through intensive training, we adapt our visual systems and attune them to recognizing letters and words from a series of black squiggles to then connect that visual input to our linguistic brain systems, a theory that has been referred to as the "neuronal recycling hypothesis" (Dehaene and Cohen, "Cultural Recycling of Cortical Maps" 384). This hypothesis, which postulates that we reuse existing brain circuits to accommodate cultural inventions such as reading, is backed up by evidence showing that learning to read and write modifies our neural networks.

After light hits the page and reflects patterns into the retina, this information is conveyed to the visual cortex. The visual cortex, in the brain's occipital lobe, breaks the image sent to the retina down into its basic elements – lines, orientation, contrast – to then recombine them in further stages to convey their shapes. For those people who have learned to read, experiments in functional neuroimaging have consistently reported an area in the left occipitotemporal cortex that shows preferential activation for letters and words over any other type of visual stimuli, such as line drawings, faces, or landscapes (Jobard et al.). This area has been called the *visual word form area* or the *brain's letterbox* (Dehaene and Cohen, "Unique Role"); it picks up the black shapes, detects the features that correspond to each letter – regardless of calligraphy or typography variations – and has more connections to the brain linguistic systems that any other area in the visual cortex.

Once the visual word form area has recognized the letters that form words on a page or screen, this information will continue to be processed in two parallel nervous pathways. The *phonological route*, through which the letter strings are transformed into sounds, involves the superior regions of the left temporal lobe, which include the auditory cortex and other regions important for speech analysis, but also some prefrontal cortices, part of the motor system, which are involved in articulation, including Broca's area. This pathway, where visual letters and spoken sounds meet, accounts for the "inner voice" we hear in our heads when reading.

On the other hand, through the *lexical route*, the orthographic units are recognized as a single word and tied to the *mental lexicon*, to then be associated with its meaning or semantics. The brain networks responsible for this process begin in the middle and anterior portions of the temporal lobe (near the classic Wernicke's area). Research has shown that portions of these areas of the temporal lobe are subdivided into regions that respond preferentially to different categories of words, both in the more general sense – nouns or verbs – and in more fine-grained distinctions, such as words referring to living versus non-living things including faces, people, animals, and edible things (Beauchamp et al.; Chao et al.). These brain areas in the temporal lobe seem to act like routers for each word's meaning, identifying which broader category it belongs to and then guiding the connections to other areas that code for the word's specific properties. But the brain's *semantic network* – described in more detail in the next section – goes beyond the temporal lobe. Research has shown that the activations in the brain induced by different words are widespread and complex, with every word activating a particular pattern of distributed brain regions, including sensorimotor areas of the brain that are related to the properties and the ways we interact with each word's referent (Dehaene).

## Meaning in the Brain: A Case for Embodied Semantics

All the neural operations described above are performed subconsciously. Our nervous systems extract shapes from light and dark patterns, recognize letters, put them together, and tie them to their sound and to their general semantic category without our knowledge or care. All we get when reading, as a result, is what we perceive as immediate access to words' sound and meaning.

How meaning is encoded in our neural circuits has been the subject of debates in philosophy and cognitive science even before neuroimaging techniques started offering windows into the semantic brain. The more classical, cognitivist view of language considered that language existed in our mind's system of purely abstract learned symbols, placing more emphasis on their interrelationships that on what they designate, and suggesting our minds can manipulate and recombine these symbols without any obvious relationship to their referent in the world, like computers do (Lloyd and Fodor; Pylyshyn). But tying symbols to other symbols – imagine, for example, trying to learn the definition of a word by looking for it in the dictionary, only to find a string made of other words that we have to look for again, finding another string of words, and so forth – would lead us to an endless loop of meaningless tokens (Vincent-Lamarre et al.). This endless circle of definitions can be broken only by words whose meanings we already know by some means other than verbal definition. This is the "symbol grounding problem" (Harnad); according to it, to generate useful behaviour, at least some symbols must be tied to their referents in the external world.

The way we, as humans, connect words to their referents in the world is through the body, by receiving and filtering information through the senses and interacting with objects, situations, and places until we understand what is what and what to do with what (or in what situation). This process, through which we learn new categories (or concepts) goes beyond just naming things: we need to abstract the essential features (sensory properties and forms of interaction) of things in the world and discard irrelevant details and infinite singularities to organize the world around us in significant groups towards which we can act in a meaningful way (Pérez-Gay Juárez et al.). After having grounded a set of symbols (words) this way, the power of language lies in its "recombinatorial" capacity: once a few words make sense, we can use them in different ways to explain the meaning of new words and use these new words in turn to create other meanings, not only by uttering straight definitions but also by telling stories. As a result, we don't need to interact with every possible entity in the world to connect the symbols with their referents, just a few that we can use to define the rest.

In line with these ideas, "embodied theories of semantics" (Barsalou; Meteyard et al.) argue that sensory and motor information are a necessary part of meaning acquisition and retrieval. The idea behind this is that when we learn a word through experience, our linguistic and sensorimotor brain networks are co-activated, generating shared neural circuits that will be later involved in semantic retrieval (Pulvermüller). When we hear, for example, the word *apple*, our mind evokes different features that are common across apples: their roundness, their sweetness, their colour, and the way we interact with an apple – how we hold it in our hands and bite it. Neuroscientific research has generated empirical evidence that retrieving the meaning of a word does imply the activation of neural circuits that respond to different modalities of information; in the case of the word *apple*, hearing or reading the word will induce activation of the visual cortex in the occipital lobe for its shape and colour properties, of the motor cortex in the frontal lobe for the movements we do when we bite it, and of the gustatory cortices in the insular lobe for its taste (Boulenger et al.; González et al.). In turn, a hand-related verb such as *grab* or *pinch* will activate the motor cortex and, to be more specific, the part of the motor cortex we use to move our hand in real life (Hauk et al.).

These studies that have shown "fragments of meaning" (Dehaene 39), distributed over the whole surface of the brain, active as soon as 200 milliseconds after the presentation of a word (Mollo et al.), provide empirical evidence to support that, at least in the case of concrete concepts, sensory and motor areas of the brain encode at least part of word semantics (Meteyard et al.; Hauk and Tschentscher). In the brain, the circuits that are active when we perceive and interact with things and situations are at least partially active when listening to or reading the words that name them, suggesting an overlap between the perceptual and conceptual circuits of the brain (Borghesani and Piazza). Whether this is the case for abstract words is still a subject of debate. Nevertheless, there is some empirical evidence suggesting that abstract words can activate motor and sensory brain circuits (Dreyer and Pulvermüller). According to some proponents of embodied semantic theories, perception and action processes in the brain also guide the construction of abstract concepts, even if the mapping between the word's features or properties and the activation in brain's sensorimotor cortices are not as obvious as they are with concrete words (Goldstone and Barsalou).

In any case, the neuroscientific and neuropsychological evidence for meaning "embodiment" should set a solid basis to go beyond the way the brain processes single words and discuss two relevant concepts in narrative engagement: *imagery* and *simulation*.

## Narratives as Model Making: Stories, Transportation, and Simulation

Real-life linguistic exercises – from trivial conversations to reading or telling intricate stories – go beyond single-word recognition. The evidence for engagement of sensory and motor systems when processing language described above has also been found in subjects who are reading stories, suggesting that these "embodiment" phenomena described for reading single words are also present when engaging with larger linguistic structures, such as narratives. In one study, researchers pre-identified the segments of a narrative that depicted different types of events – changes in location, interactions with objects, changes in temporal reference and goal setting by characters in the narrative. Subjects were then asked to read the story while inside a functional brain imaging scanner. The results from the study showed activation of the brain areas that process this type of situation in real life (frontal hand-related motor areas when a character grasps and pulls a light cord; temporal lobe areas related to scene recognition when characters change location, and so forth), and these activations were linked to story comprehension, suggesting that readers understand stories by "simulating" the narrated events (Speer et al.) and creating situation models beyond single-word and sentence recognition. According to this line of research, the coherence of these situation models within an ordered sequence is what allows for narrative comprehension.

Beyond mere comprehension, stories have the power to transport us, to create immersive experiences in which we are, even if for brief moments, absorbed from our daily lives into the narrative world (Green and Brock) in a similar way to what Csikszentmihalyi has called "flow," a state of being totally engaged in what one is doing. According to Melanie Green ("Transportation into Narrative Worlds"), narrative transportation and immersion, which could account for Coleridge's famous "suspension of disbelief" (Barad) are related to imagery, simulation, and affective processes. But what exactly do we refer to in terms of the brain when we speak about *simulation*, *imagery*, and *model making*?

In cognitive science, *imagery* refers to the creation or recreation of experience involving sensorial, perceptual or affective characteristics without sensory input coming from a direct external stimulus (Nanay; Pearson et al.). This can happen spontaneously, when we engage in mind-wandering that involves memory and imagination, or it can be prompted by an external cue other than the actual stimulus, as in the case of language. In the more classic view, imagery was mostly linked to sensory properties: visual, spatial, auditory. Even in the case of imagined movement, in what was referred to as "motor imagery," it referred to bodily sensation and not to actual motor commands (Moulton and Kosslyn). The "motor simulation theory" (Jeannerod) challenged this view, suggesting that motor imagery also involves some degree of activation of the brain's regions that we use to move. Soon, there was enough behavioural, neuropsychological, and neuroscientific evidence to support that, as described above for reading, imagining ourselves or other people moving recruits motor brain networks without producing overt movement. These networks include the premotor and supplementary motor areas – related to movement planning – as well as the primary motor cortex and some subcortical structures such as the basal ganglia, related to movement execution and control, and their activation points to a biological basis to understand motor imagery as action simulation (Hardwick et al.)

This activation of the motor system in the absence of overt movement is an example of the *simulation* or *mental enactments* that happen in our mind when we engage in narratives. Within this phenomenon, special emphasis has been given to the "mirror neuron mechanisms" that not only encompass motor simulation but are also tied to emotional recognition and empathy (Gallese and Goldman). Since the discovery of mirror neurons –neurons in the premotor cortex that are active both when we execute a motor act and when we observe another individual performing the same act (Rizzolatti et al.) – neuroscientific studies have confirmed that understanding and learning do not need the direct execution of movement but that they can be achieved through simulation, triggered by observation, imagination, or linguistic expressions (Gallese and Sinigaglia; Kim et al.). Interestingly, mirror neuron mechanisms do not only simulate actions but also seem to convey understanding beyond the actions we observe or imagine. Mirroring has been found to happen when we read other's facial expressions – if someone smiles, you smile back, and then you recognize, through your own smile, that the other person may be feeling joy. By activating our own comparable experience and expression of emotion, we can recognize what others feel. This response has also been found when reading words that indicate emotional expressions, suggesting that recognition of emotions in literary characters also involves mirroring (Foroni and Semin; Oatley, *Such Stuff as Dreams*). In this way, reading and understanding stories is making our own version (or "model") of the action in the story, gaining access to the motives behind it. This has been postulated as the basis of *narrative empathy*, defined as the "the sharing of feeling and perspective-taking induced by reading, viewing, hearing, or imagining narratives of another's situation and condition" (Keen 521) and may be an important part of the flow of emotion we experience when we go through a narrative sequence of events.

In line with these ideas, it has been shown that those who identify more with characters in a story tend to feel more transported while reading it (Green, "Transportation into Narrative Worlds: The Role of Prior Knowledge"; Johnson). Interestingly, one recent study looking at the brain's connections while reading a story showed that stronger narrative transportation was linked to higher indices of connectivity between the anterior insula, which is important to analyzing bodily reactions and emotional experiences, to sensory and motor cortices, suggesting that immersion in a story generates an integration of sensorimotor and affective information in the brain (Vaccaro et al.). Moreover, this study confirms previous findings showing that sensorimotor and emotional simulation while reading a story are linked to the activity of brain networks related to mind-wandering and self-referential thought: the default mode network. This set of interconnected brain regions is normally active when we are not engaging in a specific task but rather are involved in a number of different processes that include autobiographical memory, imaginative thinking of the future, and perspective taking (Spreng et al.; Vaccaro et al.). Through all these processes, literary fiction offers a perfect venue to create "mental models" (Craik; Oatley, *Such Stuff as Dreams*) that allow us to experience worlds that are not present, engaging in self-directed thought and introspection, learning about our own beliefs, and gaining emotional awareness.

## Fiction and Perspective Taking: Simulation of Social Worlds

When we read fiction, we are presented with scenarios in a setting in which we are not expected to react. Some authors have suggested that this disengagement from the need to initiate behaviour through movement execution (achieved through the signals from the motor cortex to the muscles), allows sensorimotor and affective systems behind imagery and simulation to reconnect with other brain areas and serve newly cognitive skills, such as understanding others (Oatley, "Fiction: Simulation of Social Worlds"; Wojciehowski and Gallese). In fact, one of the best scientifically documented effects of reading fiction is its potential to increase understanding of other people's mental states – emotions, motivations, beliefs – an ability known as theory of mind (Premack and Woodruff), mentalizing, or mind-reading.

Theory of mind (ToM) is a core component of social cognition closely related to empathy, critical to our social behaviours. Even holding a simple conversation or interpreting a stranger's relatively simple actions (entering a room, staring, and then storming out) requires making assumptions about the beliefs and intentions of the other person, which are not directly attainable by us. When engaging with fictional narratives, we construct an active model of what is going on, where we can emotionally engage with characters, reflect about their motives, and imagine possible outcomes of their actions without the need of an immediate behavioural reaction. In this way, narratives provide a protected, parallel space in which to perform mental experiments about social cognition (Mar and Oatley) and moral dilemmas (Bacha-Trams et al.; Hakemulder). Through this process, fiction has for a long time been believed to improve social cognition, namely two interrelated phenomena: empathy and ToM.

ToM and empathy are sometimes presented as complementary, with empathy representing emotional perspective taking (in which we vicariously experience the emotion of others) while ToM represents cognitive perspective taking (in which we understand and recognize the emotion of others) (Hynes et al.). Others classify the former as emotional or affective empathy and the latter as cognitive empathy (Decety and Jackson; Shamay-Tsoory et al.). In terms of the brain, the first one is more closely associated with the mirroring processes described in the previous section, while the second appears to engage other higher order cognitive processes such as language and executive functions (Meinhardt-Injac et al.), which allow us to separate belief from fact, understand causality, and engage in moral reasoning (Healey and Grossman). In any case, these two processes, even if they can be behaviourally and neurally dissociated, are integrated to serve the same final function: taking a different point of view to make sense of others (Maibom), a crucial skill to navigate the complexity of our social lives.

Fiction reading provides an ideal scenario in which to exercise perspective taking, for it allows us to plunge into the inner life of characters and discover their hidden motives, beliefs, and emotions, which enables us to have a better understanding of their actions than from merely observing their behaviour (Oatley, "Fiction: Simulation of Social Worlds"). Frank Hakemulder has referred to the novel as a "moral laboratory" in which we can freely experience and analyze scenarios that we would not have encountered otherwise. Oatley, in turn, refers to fiction as a "simulation of social worlds" or even as a form of consciousness that can be passed from one mind to another. This idea of simulation goes beyond the sensorimotor or mirroring simulations described above; it comprises more abstract representations orchestrated by the association cortices of the brain, including creating a model of others' mental states, for which we need, at least for a moment, to disengage from our own perspective. This is why Lisa Zunshine has proposed that ToM, or perspective taking, is probably the central enterprise in fiction reading.

Recently, neuroimaging studies have shed light on the neural bases of this improvement in social cognition. Similarly to the studies that showed activation in sensorimotor brain areas when reading about subjects performing actions or sensory-rich descriptions of scenarios, reading about fictional characters activates the brain regions that we use when interacting in our real social world, the so called "mentalizing brain networks" (Oatley, "Fiction: Simulation of Social Worlds"). After performing a meta-analysis of the neuroimaging data, Mars et al. showed that regions that are active in the mentalizing network overlap with those in the default mode network described above. The authors interpret these findings to suggest that we use mind-wandering to analyze issues related to our dynamic social world, which are central to our growth and survival. The finding that reading fiction activates mentalizing networks confirms that social cognition is also central in our fiction-induced simulations and suggests that our nervous systems treat fictional characters in a similar way as people in our lives (Mar; Spreng et al.; Summerfield et al.; Tamir et al.). Guided by the writer, who provides us with more details about what goes on in the characters' minds than we would be able to access in real life, fiction trains our social brains by making us simulate interactions with remarkably diverse characters and situations.

Correlational studies studying the effect of lifelong reading habits on social cognition seem to support the idea that fiction trains our social abilities. Lifetime fiction reading has, for example, been correlated with stronger affective empathy and helping tendencies (Stansfield and Bunce), with a significantly larger correlation measure than non-fiction reading (Mumper and Gerrig). This association between reading habits, empathy, and ToM has been found not to depend on more empathetic people preferring to read fiction and remained after controlling for personality and other individual differences (Mar et al.). Going further, accumulating evidence shows that inducing perspective taking through fiction reading (e.g., in an experimental setting) can causally impact social cognition, leading to a significant improvement in socio-cognitive performance, including ToM, while not leading to improved performance on cognitive tasks overall (Dodell-Feder and Tamir; Kidd and Castano, "Reading Improves Theory of Mind"; Kidd and Catsano, "Three Pre-Registered Replications"). The evidence suggests that the length of the text also influences the strength of this effect, and the study in which participants read an entire book led to one of the largest effect sizes (Pino and Mazza). When it comes to medium-term impacts of reading, one study found that participants were more empathetic one week after having read a story if they had been emotionally involved in it (Bal and Veltkamp). In another, fiction reading prompted empathy and reflection in the days after reading (Koopman).

Researchers in the field have identified two interrelated ways in which fiction could train social cognition. The first is the *process way*, which goes back to the idea of fiction as a simulation: by imagining story characters and their mental state, fiction reading trains our perspective-taking abilities and provides readers with additional practice on the social processes that are used during real-world interactions (Oatley, "Fiction: Simulation of Social Worlds"). This mechanism emphasizes that the usefulness of fiction reading cannot be reduced to its content but is also due to the literary form. This is supported by a large literature that has attempted to disentangle the effect of the literariness of a text from other features (like its fictionality) on its impact on social cognition, notably by comparing the effect of reading literary or high-brow fiction to that of reading popular fiction (Schwerin and Lenhart). Recently, Castano et al. have confirmed that different types of fiction have divergent effects on social cognition: exposure to literature fiction (which can be considered of higher literariness) is, for example, associated with better performance in tests of ToM, while popular fiction is negatively associated with attributional complexity, a construct which measures how complexly we think about the causes of others' behaviours. This difference may occur because literature fiction, with its emphasis on the characters rather than the scenario, forces the readers to consider a higher number of complex perspectives than does popular fiction. It could also be linked to findings that higher transportation can induce higher social changes, such as reduced prejudicial attitudes (Mazzocco et al.) and that transportation depends on the degree of imagery, which is conveyed by – and related to – literary form.

In this view, the degree of transportation will have an effect on the extent to which we make models of what others are thinking or feeling.

One important thing to note is that while the content of literature can be used to reduce prejudice and bias between social groups, pieces of literature that feature racist, sexist, or otherwise discriminatory content can – without surprise – have the opposite effect. Similarly, the impact of the literary form on social cognition does not necessarily lead to positive change in terms of social justice and equity. Indeed, a person can be made to empathize with and gain a better understanding of any type of characters, and in certain contexts such understanding can be used to support narratives that legitimize systemic structures of violences, such as settler colonialism. In our opinion, it is not merely reading literary fiction but engaging with narratives from *diverse social groups* – including narratives from marginalized groups and minorities – which can, through the neurocognitive mechanisms suggested above, help us generate empathy and understanding of others, providing a strategy to reduce prejudice, discrimination, and perceptions of "otherness." Therefore, this chapter does not intend to suggest that reading fiction per se will result in overcoming systemic structures of violence, inequity, and racism. Rather, we aim to provide a cognitive science background to understand how and why literary fiction stimulates perspective taking and social cognition processes.

The other way through which fiction could influence social cognition is through its *content*: by providing more specific information about human psychology, social interaction, or distinct cultures and people that readers might not have access to otherwise, fiction reading can increase the social knowledge of readers (Mar and Oatley). This is of utmost relevance for researchers who, like the authors of this chapter, are interested in the way reading fiction can help reduce biases and improve empathy towards people outside our social groups, including members of marginalized or stigmatized communities. Research in social psychology shows that higher contact with members of other social groups can increase empathy and decrease stereotyping and discrimination (Kubota et al.). However, there is a certain limit to the number of people we can interact with and promoting social contact with members of other groups may not always be feasible nor comfortable for the people involved. Literary fiction, in contrast, provides an ideal scenario to engage in simulated contact in a safe space, challenging readers' biases as they explore the perspective of people with whom they would not normally interact. In fact, some experimental studies have already started to show the potential of fiction to reduce prejudice and bias towards minority groups (Johnson; Johnson et al.; Vezzali et al., "Greatest Gift"; Vezzali et al., "May the Odds"). This, of course, highlights the importance of engaging with fiction whose *content* includes the perspectives of characters that are diverse in terms of culture, gender, sexuality, and mental health.

### Fiction and Well-Being: A Necessary Dialogue between Literary Arts, Health Humanities, and Neuroscience

The evidence summarized so far suggests that, when we read about fictional situations, our nervous systems show similar patterns of activity as they do when we encounter those situations in real life, suggesting that the border between real and fictional worlds in our minds is less sharp than we previously thought (Gallese; Oatley, "Fiction: Simulation of Social Worlds"). On the other hand, immersion in fictional narratives offers a venue of disconnection from our presence in daily life, which allows us to explore and test models of situations and people we may never encounter in real life in a parallel, protected space. In this way, literary fiction induces simulations in our brains that connect those models to aspects of our own selves, helping us recognize what goes "beyond the surface" (Oatley, *Such Stuff as Dreams*) and perform mental experiments about social cognition and moral dilemmas. In the same way that learning to read modifies our existing brain circuits, there is neuroscientific evidence showing that reading fiction and engaging with literary narratives can also modify our nervous system and our psychological world and therefore our understanding and behaviour.

Recent collaborations between neuroscientists, artists and scholars in the humanities have given rise to "neurohumanism," which includes cognitive poetics, cognitive historicism, cognitive film studies, and cognitive cultural studies (Frazzeto and Anker) and "neuroaesthetics" (Zeki). In parallel, different lines of scientific research have started to delve into the importance of the arts for the benefit of mental health, human dignity, and well-being, supporting the transformative power of artistic practices, long known in the arts and the humanities fields but relatively ignored or underestimated in the biomedical field. The quantitative biological evidence of the benefits of reading literary fiction offered by cognitive neuroscience has the potential to permeate into the biomedical model, while its different perspectives – mostly related to 4E (embodied, embedded, extended, and enactive) cognition (Gallagher) – leave room for the interaction between biology and sociocultural contexts that are of utmost relevance for health humanities. Through this lens, we aim to move beyond biological and cultural determinism to open a dialogue that allows us to address, as William Conolly has put it in his work introducing the field of neuropolitics, "how biology is mixed into thinking and culture and how other aspects of nature are folded into both." We believe that bringing attention to these aspects of the cognitive neuroscience of fiction will help this transdisciplinary exchange, hoping to (1) provide neurobiological data to shape or inspire literary creation and intervention, (2) broadcast the potential of fiction to tackle social issues such as discrimination and stigma towards minorities, and (3) open a window for standard psychological and medical narratives to look towards literary arts as venues to improve wellbeing and mental health.

## WORKS CITED

Bacha-Trams, Mareike, et al. "Differential Inter-Subject Correlation of Brain Activity When Kinship Is a Variable in Moral Dilemma." *Scientific Reports*, vol. 7, no. 1, Oct. 2017, pp. 1–16, https://doi.org/10.1038/s41598-017-14323-x.

Bal, P. Matthijs, and Martijn Veltkamp. "How Does Fiction Reading Influence Empathy? An Experimental Investigation on the Role of Emotional Transportation." *PLOS ONE*, vol. 8, no. 1, Jan. 2013, Article e55341, https://doi.org/10.1371/JOURNAL.PONE.0055341.

Baldassano, Christopher, et al. "Representation of Real-World Event Schemas during Narrative Perception." *Journal of Neuroscience*, vol. 38, no. 45, Nov. 2018, pp. 9689–99, https://doi.org/10.1523/JNEUROSCI.0251-18.2018.

Barad, Dilip. "Sanuel Taylor Coleridge – Biographia Literaria: Ch14." *Teacher Blog*, 6 Oct. 2015, https://blog.dilipbarad.com/2015/10/coleridge-biographia-literaria.html.

Barsalou, Lawrence W. "Perceptual Symbol Systems." *Behavioraland Brain Sciences*, vol. 22, no. 4, 1999, pp. 577–660, https://doi.org/10.1017/S0140525X99002149.

Bassett, Danielle S., and Olaf Sporns. "Network Neuroscience." *Nature Neuroscience*, vol. 20, no. 3, Feb. 2017, p. 353, https://doi.org/10.1038/NN.4502.

Beauchamp, Michael S., et al. "Integration of Auditory and Visual Information about Objects in Superior Temporal Sulcus." *Neuron*, vol. 41, no. 5, Mar. 2004, pp. 809–23, https://doi.org/10.1016/S0896-6273(04)00070-4/ATTACHMENT/EE0D2F98-5111-49F0-8044-881C176C773D/MMC1.PDF.

Binder, Jeffrey R. "The Wernicke Area: Modern Evidence and a Reinterpretation." *Neurology*, vol. 85, no. 24, Dec. 2015, p. 2170, https://doi.org/10.1212/WNL.0000000000002219.

Borghesani, Valentina, and Manuela Piazza. "The Neuro-Cognitive Representations of Symbols: The Case of Concrete Words." *Neuropsychologia*, vol. 105, Oct. 2017, pp. 4–17, https://doi.org/10.1016/J.NEUROPSYCHOLOGIA.2017.06.026.

Boulenger, Véronique, et al. "Grasping Ideas with the Motor System: Semantic Somatotopy in Idiom Comprehension." *Cerebral Cortex*, vol. 19, no. 8, Aug. 2009, pp. 1905–14, https://doi.org/10.1093/CERCOR/BHN217.

Castano, Emanuele, et al. "The Effect of Exposure to Fiction on Attributional Complexity, Egocentric Bias and Accuracy in Social Perception." *PLOS ONE*, vol. 15, no. 5, 2020, Article e0233378, https://doi.org/10.1371/journal.pone.0233378.

Chao, Linda L., et al. "Attribute-Based Neural Substrates in Temporal Cortex for Perceiving and Knowing about Objects." *Nature Neuroscience*, vol. 2, no. 10, Oct. 1999, pp. 913–19, https://doi.org/10.1038/13217.

Chomsky, Noam. *Syntactic Structures*. Martino Publishing, 2015.

Connolly, William E. *Neuropolitics: Thinking, Culture, Speed*. U of Minnesota P, 2002.

Craik, Kenneth. *The Nature of Explanation*. Cambridge UP, 1943.

Csikszentmihalyi, Mihaly. *Flow: The Psychology of Optimal Experience*. Harper & Row, 1990.

Decety, Jean, and Philip L. Jackson. "The Functional Architecture of Human Empathy." *Behavioraland Cognitive Neuroscience Reviews*, vol. 3, no. 2, 2004, pp. 71–100, https://doi.org/10.1177/1534582304267187.

Dehaene, Stanislas. *Reading in the Brain: The New Science of How We Read*. Penguin Books, 2010.

Dehaene, Stanislas, and Laurent Cohen. "Cultural Recycling of Cortical Maps." *Neuron*, vol. 56, no. 2, Oct. 2007, pp. 384–98, https://doi.org/10.1016/J.NEURON.2007.10.004.

–. "The Unique Role of the Visual Word Form Area in Reading." *Trends in Cognitive Sciences*, vol. 15, no. 6, June 2011, pp. 254–62, https://doi.org/10.1016/J.TICS.2011.04.003.

Dehaene-Lambertz, Ghislaine, et al. "Functional Organization of Perisylvian Activation during Presentation of Sentences in Preverbal Infants." *Proceedings of the National Academy of Sciences of the United States of America*, vol. 103, no. 38, Sept. 2006, p. 14240–45. https://doi.org/10.1073/PNAS.0606302103.

Dodell-Feder, David, and Diana I. Tamir. "Fiction Reading Has a Small Positive Impact on Social Cognition: A Meta-Analysis." *Journal of Experimental Psychology: General*, vol. 147, no. 11, Nov. 2018, pp. 1713–27, https://doi.org/10.1037/XGE0000395.

Dreyer, Felix R., and Friedemann Pulvermüller. "Abstract Semantics in the Motor System? – An Event-Related FMRI Study on Passive Reading of Semantic Word Categories Carrying Abstract Emotional and Mental Meaning." *Cortex*, vol. 100, Mar. 2018, pp. 52–70, https://doi.org/10.1016/J.CORTEX.2017.10.021.

Eimas, Peter D., et al. "Speech Perception in Infants." *Science*, vol. 171, no. 3968, 1971, pp. 303–6, https://doi.org/10.1126/SCIENCE.171.3968.303.

Foroni, Francesco, and Gün R. Semin. "Language That Puts You in Touch with Your Bodily Feelings: The Multimodal Responsiveness of Affective Expressions." *Psychological Science*, vol. 20, no. 8, Aug. 2009, pp. 974–80, https://doi.org/10.1111/j.1467-9280.2009.02400.x.

Frazzetto, Giovanni, and Suzanne Anker. "Neuroculture." *Nature Reviews. Neuroscience*, vol. 10, no. 11, 2009, pp. 815–21. https://doi.org/10.1038/nrn2736.

Gallagher, M. "4E Cognition and the Spectrum of Aesthetic Experience." *JOLMA. The Journal for the Philosophy of Language, Mind and the Arts*, vol. 1, no. 2, 2020, pp. 157–76, https://doi.org/10.30687/Jolma/2723-9640/2020/02/001.

Gallese, Vittorio. "Embodied Simulation Theory: Imagination and Memory." *Neuropsychoanalysis*, vol. 13, no. 2, 2011, pp. 196–200, https://doi.org/10.1080/15294145.2011.10773675.

Gallese, Vittorio, and Alvin Goldman. "Mirror Neurons and the Simulation Theory of Mind-Reading." *Trends in Cognitive Sciences*, vol. 2, no. 12, Dec. 1998, pp. 493–501, https://doi.org/10.1016/S1364-6613(98)01262-5.

Gallese, Vittorio, and Corrado Sinigaglia. "What Is So Special about Embodied Simulation?" *Trends in Cognitive Sciences*, vol. 15, no. 11, 2011, pp. 512–19, https://doi.org/10.1016/J.TICS.2011.09.003.

Goldstone, Robert L., and Lawrence W. Barsalou. "Reuniting Perception and Conception." *Cognition*, vol. 65, no. 2–3, Jan. 1998, pp. 231–62, https://doi.org/10.1016/S0010-0277(97)00047-4.

González, Julio, et al. "Reading Cinnamon Activates Olfactory Brain Regions." *NeuroImage*, vol. 32, no. 2, Aug. 2006, pp. 906–12, https://doi.org/10.1016/J.NEUROIMAGE.2006.03.037.

Green, Melanie C. "Transportation into Narrative Worlds: The Role of Prior Knowledge and Perceived Realism." *The Effects of Personal Involvement in Narrative Discourse: A Special Issue of Discourse Processes*, May 2014, pp. 247–66, https://doi.org/10.1207/S15326950DP3802_5.

–. "Transportation into Narrative Worlds." *Entertainment-Education Behind the Scenes*, 2021, pp. 87–101, https://doi.org/10.1007/978-3-030-63614-2_6.

Green, Melanie C., and Timothy C. Brock. "The Role of Transportation in the Persuasiveness of Public Narratives." *Journal of Personality and Social Psychology*, vol. 79, no. 5, 2000, pp. 701–21, https://doi.org/10.1037/0022-3514.79.5.701.

Hakemulder, J. *The Moral Laboratory*. Vol. 34, John Benjamins Publishing Company, 2000, https://doi.org/10.1075/upal.34.

Hardwick, Robert M., et al. "Neural Correlates of Action: Comparing Meta-Analyses of Imagery, Observation, and Execution." *Neuroscience and Biobehavioral Reviews*, vol. 94, Nov. 2018, pp. 31–44, https://doi.org/10.1016/J.NEUBIOREV.2018.08.003.

Harnad, Stevan. "The Symbol Grounding Problem." *Physica D: Nonlinear Phenomena*, vol. 42, no. 1–3, June 1990, pp. 335–46, https://doi.org/10.1016/0167-2789(90)90087-6.

Hauk, Olaf, et al. "Somatotopic Representation of Action Words in Human Motor and Premotor Cortex." *Neuron*, vol. 41, no. 2, Jan. 2004, pp. 301–07, https://doi.org/10.1016/S0896-6273(03)00838-9.

Hauk, Olaf, and Nadja Tschentscher. "The Body of Evidence: What Can Neuroscience Tell Us about Embodied Semantics." *Frontiers in Psychology*, vol. 4, no. Feb., 2013, https://doi.org/10.3389/FPSYG.2013.00050.

Healey, Meghan L., and Murray Grossman. "Cognitive and Affective Perspective-Taking: Evidence for Shared and Dissociable Anatomical

Substrates." *Frontiers in Neurology*, vol. 9, June 2018, Article 491, https://doi.org/10.3389/FNEUR.2018.00491.

Hertrich, Ingo, et al. "The Margins of the Language Network in the Brain." *Frontiers in Communication*, vol. 5, 2020, Article 519955, https://doi.org/10.3389/FCOMM.2020.519955.

Hickok, Gregory, et al. "The Role of Broca's Area in Speech Perception: Evidence from Aphasia Revisited." *Brain and Language*, vol. 119, no. 3, Dec. 2011, pp. 214–20, https://doi.org/10.1016/J.BANDL.2011.08.001.

Hynes, Catherine A., et al. "Differential Role of the Orbital Frontal Lobe in Emotional versus Cognitive Perspective-Taking." *Neuropsychologia*, vol. 44, no. 3, 2006, pp. 374–83, https://doi.org/10.1016/J.NEUROPSYCHOLOGIA.2005.06.011.

Imada, Toshiaki, et al. "Infant Speech Perception Activates Broca's Area: A Developmental Magnetoencephalography Study." *Neuroreport*, vol. 17, no. 10, June 2006, pp. 957–62, https://doi.org/10.1097/01.WNR.0000223387.51704.89.

Jeannerod, Marc. "Neural Simulation of Action: A Unifying Mechanism for Motor Cognition." *NeuroImage*, vol. 14, no. 1 Pt 2, 2001, https://doi.org/10.1006/NIMG.2001.0832.

Jobard, G., et al. "Evaluation of the Dual Route Theory of Reading: A Metanalysis of 35 Neuroimaging Studies." *NeuroImage*, vol. 20, no. 2, Oct. 2003, pp. 693–712, https://doi.org/10.1016/S1053-8119(03)00343-4.

Johnson, Dan R. "Transportation into a Story Increases Empathy, Prosocial Behavior, and Perceptual Bias toward Fearful Expressions." *Personality and Individual Differences*, vol. 52, no. 2, Jan. 2012, pp. 150–55, https://doi.org/10.1016/J.PAID.2011.10.005.

Johnson, Dan R., et al. "Changing Race Boundary Perception by Reading Narrative Fiction." *Basic and Applied Social Psychology*, vol. 36, no. 1, Jan. 2014, pp. 83–90, https://doi.org/10.1080/01973533.2013.856791.

Kandel, Eric. "The New Science of Mind and the Future of Knowledge." *Neuron*, vol. 80, no. 3, Oct. 2013, pp. 546–60, https://doi.org/10.1016/J.NEURON.2013.10.039.

Keen, Suzanne. "Narrative Empathy." *Handbook of Narratology*, edited by Peter Hühn et al., De Gruyter, 2014, pp. 521–30, https://doi.org/10.1515/9783110316469.521.

Keller, Simon S., et al. "Broca's Area: Nomenclature, Anatomy, Typology and Asymmetry." *Brain and Language*, vol. 109, no. 1, Apr. 2009, pp. 29–48, https://doi.org/10.1016/J.BANDL.2008.11.005.

Kidd, David, and Emanuele Castano. "Reading Literary Fiction and Theory of Mind: Three Preregistered Replications and Extensions of Kidd and Castano (2013)." *Social Psychological and Personality Science*, vol. 10, no. 4, 2019, pp. 522–31, https://doi.org/10.1177/1948550618775410.

Kidd, David Comer, and Emanuele Castano. "Reading Literary Fiction Improves Theory of Mind." *Science*, vol. 342, no. 6156, 2013, pp. 377–80, https://doi.org/10.1126/SCIENCE.1239918.

Kim, Olivia A., et al. "Motor Learning without Movement." *Proceedings of the National Academy of Sciences of the United States of America*, vol. 119, no. 30, July 2022, https://doi.org/10.1073/PNAS.2204379119.

Koopman, Eva Maria. "How Texts about Suffering Trigger Reflection: Genre, Personal Factors, and Affective Responses." *Psychology of Aesthetics, Creativity, and the Arts*, vol. 9, no. 4, Nov. 2015, pp. 430–41, https://doi.org/10.1037/ACA0000006.

Kubota, Jennifer T., et al. "Intergroup Contact throughout the Lifespan Modulates Implicit Racial Biases across Perceivers' Racial Group." *PLOS ONE*, vol. 12, no. 7, July 2017, Article e0180440, https://doi.org/10.1371/JOURNAL.PONE.0180440.

Kuhl, Patricia K. "Brain Mechanisms in Early Language Acquisition." *Neuron*, vol. 67, no. 5, Sept. 2010, pp. 713–27, https://doi.org/10.1016/J.NEURON.2010.08.038.

Kuhl, Patricia K., and Andrew N. Meltzoff. "Infant Vocalizations in Response to Speech: Vocal Imitation and Developmental Change." *Journal of the Acoustical Society of America*, vol. 100, no. 4 Pt 1, Oct. 1996, pp. 2425–38, https://doi.org/10.1121/1.417951.

Lieberman, Philip. *The Biology and Evolution of Language*. Harvard UP, 1984.

Lloyd, Dan, and Jerry A. Fodor. "Psychosemantics: The Problem of Meaning in the Philosophy of Mind." *The Philosophical Review*, vol. 100, no. 2, Apr. 1987, pp. 289–93, https://doi.org/10.2307/2185306.

Maibom, Heidi L. "Self-Simulation and Empathy." *Forms of Fellow Feeling: Empathy, Sympathy, Concern and Moral Agency*, edited by Neil Roughley and Thomas Schramme, Cambridge UP, Jan. 2018, pp. 109–32, https://doi.org/10.1017/9781316271698.004.

Mar, Raymond A. "The Neural Bases of Social Cognition and Story Comprehension." *Annual Review of Psychology*, vol. 62, Jan. 2011, pp. 103–34, https://doi.org/10.1146/ANNUREV-PSYCH-120709-145406.

Mar, Raymond A., and Keith Oatley. "The Function of Fiction Is the Abstraction and Simulation of Social Experience." *Perspectives on Psychological Science*, vol. 3, no. 3, May 2008, pp. 173–92, https://doi.org/10.1111/j.1745-6924.2008.00073.x.

Mar, Raymond A., et al. "Exploring the Link between Reading Fiction and Empathy: Ruling out Individual Differences and Examining Outcomes." *Communications*, vol. 34, no. 4, Dec. 2009, pp. 407–28, https://doi.org/10.1515/COMM.2009.025.

Mars, Rogier B., et al. "On the Relationship between the 'Default Mode Network' and the 'Social Brain.'" *Frontiers in Human Neuroscience*, vol. 6, June 2012, Article 189, https://doi.org/10.3389/FNHUM.2012.00189.

Mazzocco, Philip J., et al. "This Story Is Not for Everyone: Transportability and Narrative Persuasion." Social Psychological and Personality Science, vol. 1, no. 4, 2010, pp. 361–8, https://doi.org/10.1177/1948550610376600.

Meinhardt-Injac, Bozana, et al. "The Two-Systems Account of Theory of Mind: Testing the Links to Social-Perceptual and Cognitive Abilities." *Frontiers in Human Neuroscience*, vol. 12, Jan. 2018, Article 25, https://doi.org/10.3389/FNHUM.2018.00025.

Meteyard, Lotte, et al. "Coming of Age: A Review of Embodiment and the Neuroscience of Semantics." *Cortex*, vol. 48, no. 7, July 2012, pp. 788–804, https://doi.org/10.1016/J.CORTEX.2010.11.002.

Mollo, Giovanna, et al. "Movement Priming of EEG/MEG Brain Responses for Action-Words Characterizes the Link between Language and Action." *Cortex*, vol. 74, Jan. 2016, pp. 262–76, https://doi.org/10.1016/J.CORTEX.2015.10.021.

Moulton, Samuel T., and Stephen M. Kosslyn. "Imagining Predictions: Mental Imagery as Mental Emulation." *Philosophical Transactions of the Royal Society B: Biological Sciences*, vol. 364, no. 1521, May 2009, pp. 1273–80, https://doi.org/10.1098/RSTB.2008.0314.

Mumper, Micah L., and Richard J. Gerrig. "Leisure Reading and Social Cognition: A Meta-Analysis." *Psychology of Aesthetics, Creativity, and the Arts*, vol. 11, no. 1, Feb. 2016, pp. 109–20, https://doi.org/10.1037/ACA0000089.

Nanay, Bence. "Multimodal Mental Imagery." Cortex, vol. 105, 2018, pp. 125–34. https://doi.org/10.1016/j.cortex.2017.07.006

Nasios, Grigorios, et al. "From Broca and Wernicke to the Neuromodulation Era: Insights of Brain Language Networks for Neurorehabilitation." *BehaviouralNeurology*, vol. 2019, no. 1, 2019, Article 9894571, https://doi.org/10.1155/2019/9894571.

Oatley, Keith. *Such Stuff as Dreams: The Psychology of Fiction*. Wiley-Blackwell, 2011.

–. "Fiction: Simulation of Social Worlds." *Trends in Cognitive Sciences*, vol. 20, no. 8, 2016, pp. 618–28, https://doi.org/10.1016/j.tics.2016.06.002.

Pearson, Joel, et al. "Mental Imagery: Functional Mechanisms and Clinical Applications." *Trends in Cognitive Sciences*, vol. 19, no. 10, 2015, pp. 590–602, https://doi.org/10.1016/J.TICS.2015.08.003.

Pino, Maria Chiara, and Monica Mazza. "The Use of 'Literary Fiction' to Promote Mentalizing Ability." *PloS One*, vol. 11, no. 8, 2016, Article e0160254, https://doi.org/10.1371/JOURNAL.PONE.0160254.

Pérez-Gay Juárez, Fernanda, et al. "Category Learning Can Alter Perception and Its Neural Correlates." *PLoS ONE*, vol. 14, no. 12, 2019, Article e0226000, https://doi.org/10.1371/journal.pone.0226000.

Premack, David, and Guy Woodruff. "Does the Chimpanzee Have a Theory of Mind?" *Behavioraland Brain Sciences*, vol. 1, no. 4, 1978, pp. 515–26, https://doi.org/10.1017/S0140525X00076512.

Pulvermüller, Friedemann. "Words in the Brain's Language." *Behavioraland Brain Sciences*, vol. 22, no. 2, 1999, pp. 253–336, https://doi.org/10.1017/S0140525X9900182X.

Pylyshyn, Zenon W. *Computation and Cognition: Toward a Foundation for Cognitive Science*. MIT Press, 1984.

Rizzolatti, Giacomo, et al. "Premotor Cortex and the Recognition of Motor Actions." *Cognitive Brain Research*, vol. 3, no. 2, 1996, pp. 131–41, https://doi.org/10.1016/0926-6410(95)00038-0.

Schwerin, Julia, and Jan Lenhart. "The Effects of Literariness on Social-Cognitive Skills: Examining Narrative Engagement, Transportation, and Identification as Moderators." Psychology of Aesthetics, Creativity, and the Arts, vol. 19, no. 2, 2022, pp. 181–92. https://doi.org/10.1037/aca0000514.

Shamay-Tsoory, Simone G., et al. "Two Systems for Empathy: A Double Dissociation between Emotional and Cognitive Empathy in Inferior Frontal Gyrus versus Ventromedial Prefrontal Lesions." *Brain: A Journal of Neurology*, vol. 132, no. 3, 2009, pp. 617–27, https://doi.org/10.1093/BRAIN/AWN279.

Skinner, B.F. *Verbal Behavior*. Appleton-Century-Crofts, 1957.

Speer, Nicole K., et al. "Human Brain Activity Time-Locked to Narrative Event Boundaries." *Psychological Science*, vol. 18, no. 5, 2007, 449–55. https://doi.org/10.1111/j.1467-9280.2007.01920.x.

Spreng, R. Nathan, et al. "The Common Neural Basis of Autobiographical Memory, Prospection, Navigation, Theory of Mind, and the Default Mode: A Quantitative Meta-Analysis." *Journal of Cognitive Neuroscience*, vol. 21, no. 3, Mar. 2009, pp. 489–510, https://doi.org/10.1162/JOCN.2008.21029.

Stansfield, John, and Louise Bunce. "The Relationship between Empathy and Reading Fiction: Separate Roles for Cognitive and Affective Components." *Journal of European Psychology Students*, vol. 5, no. 3, July 2014, pp. 9–18, https://doi.org/10.5334/JEPS.CA.

Summerfield, Jennifer J., et al. "Differential Engagement of Brain Regions within a 'Core' Network during Scene Construction." *Neuropsychologia*, vol. 48, no. 5, Apr. 2010, pp. 1501–9, https://doi.org/10.1016/J.NEUROPSYCHOLOGIA.2010.01.022.

Tamir, Diana I., et al. "Reading Fiction and Reading Minds: The Role of Simulation in the Default Network." *Social Cognitive and Affective Neuroscience*, vol. 11, no. 2, Apr. 2016, pp. 215–24, https://doi.org/10.1093/SCAN/NSV114.

Vaccaro, Anthony G., et al. "Functional Brain Connectivity during Narrative Processing Relates to Transportation and Story Influence." *Frontiers in Human Neuroscience*, vol. 15, July 2021, Article 665319, https://doi.org/10.3389/FNHUM.2021.665319.

Vezzali, Loris, Shelley McKeown, et al. "May the Odds Be Ever in Your Favor: The Hunger Games and the Fight for a More Equal Society. (Negative)

Media Vicarious Contact and Collective Action." *Journal of Applied Social Psychology*, vol. 51, no. 2, Feb. 2021, pp. 121–37, https://doi.org/10.1111/JASP.12721.

Vezzali, Loris, Sofia Stathi, et al. "The Greatest Magic of Harry Potter: Reducing Prejudice." *Journal of Applied Social Psychology*, vol. 45, no. 2, Feb. 2015, pp. 105–21, https://doi.org/10.1111/JASP.12279.

Vincent-Lamarre, Philippe, et al. "The Latent Structure of Dictionaries." *Topics in Cognitive Science*, vol. 8, no. 3, July 2016, pp. 625–59, https://doi.org/10.1111/TOPS.12211.

Wojciehowski, Hannah, and Vittorio Gallese. "Embodiment : Embodied Simulation and Emotional Engagement With Fictional Characters." *The Routledge Companion to Literature and Emotion*, edited by Patrick Colm Hogan et al., Routledge, Feb. 2022, pp. 61–73, https://doi.org/10.4324/9780367809843-7.

Zeki, Semir, et al. "Neuroaesthetics: The Art, Science, and Brain Triptych." *PsyCh Journal*, vol. 9, no. 4, 2020, pp. 427–8. https://doi.org/10.1002/pchj.383.

Zunshine, Lisa. *Why We Read Fiction: Theory of Mind and the Novel*. Ohio State UP, 2006.

# 2 The "Villainous Obstinacy and Ugliness" of "a Body of Facts": The Creation of the Character of Alexis Saint-Martin by His Surgeon, Dr. William Beaumont

MAXIME RAYMOND BOCK

In popular culture today, *coureurs des bois* and *voyageurs* – indentured servants (or *engagés*) of mostly French Canadian origins carrying merchandise all over North America for the benefit of powerful French, English, and American fur trade companies – have been reified into folkloric clichés that provoke amused condescension, if not disdain, or outright rejection. A recent controversy in Quebec literature illustrates the contempt for these historical figures and the iconography associated with them. In 2022, among the three shortlisted novels for the Prix France-Québec, two were historical novels, *L'étonnante destinée de Pierre Boucher* by Nicole Lavigne, and *1542: La colonie maudite* by Raymond Rainville. These selections sparked heated debates in the media over the books' merits, implying that they were not qualified to represent Quebec in an international literary competition. Underlying this reaction is the fact that Quebec historical fiction in itself was not considered worthy of such a prestigious prize and must therefore remain a para-literary genre. Neither of the book jackets represented Quebec's modern identity or the vitality of its contemporary writing culture: both featured a birchbark canoe. Arguments were made that this was only a choice to appeal to the "ma cabane au Canada" trope French readers in France are notoriously fond of (Paré). But what transpired through this indignant reaction was that in the eyes of Quebecois commentators themselves, the notion that their own ancestors, who shaped the North American geopolitical economics for more than 225 years from Samuel de Champlain to the decline of the fur trade in the 1840s – when Canada itself as an official country is only 156 years old – are estranged, exotic figures.

Examples of unsympathetic French Canadian voyageur figures can also be found in recent popular movies or tv series, this time through the gaze of Mexican, American, and Canadian creators: *The Revenant*, a 2015 movie by Alejandro G. Iñárritu about the American adventurer

Hugh Glass is set in the 1820s on the Missouri River; *Frontier*, a 2016 Canadian television series about the fur trade rivalries in Hudson's Bay Company's Rupert's Land, at the turn of the nineteenth century; and *Prey*, a 2022 *Predator* franchise film set in the American Great Plains in 1719, where members of the Comanche Nation fight aliens from outer space. The three productions depict the voyageurs with the same clichés. In the *Revenant* and in *Prey*, groups of French Canadian *hommes du Nord*, or Northmen, are shown to be lawless, rowdy, uncultured, violent drunkards; in *Frontier*, the character of Jean-Marc Rivard is a not-so-intelligent French Canadian fur trader who acts as an informant between Indigenous, American, Scottish, Irish, and British interests depending on who pays him the best wages, and sometimes an extra pint of brandy – downed in a single gulp – is enough to tip the scale. What stands out from these depictions, apart from the aforementioned characteristics, is that voyageurs lack subjectivity, either because they are anonymized among an indistinct group or because they don't act of their own accord, subjected to forces that determine them, notably greed.

These enduring prejudices about French-Canadian voyageurs have been commonplace since there first were *coureurs de bois*, and for many reasons. First, the authorities of New France (1534–1760) drew a negative portrait of the tradesmen in order to prevent young men from abandoning their agricultural responsibilities in the St. Lawrence River Valley. Second, the voyageurs themselves narrated their life stories through tall tales, exaggerating feats of prowess, and a love of freedom that has since mutated in our collective imagery into a fallacious yearning for the absence of rules or hierarchy. Third, and this is the subject of this essay, the written sources about them were, in a vast majority, from writers who were not voyageurs themselves: clerks, bourgeois, rich traders from Montreal or elsewhere, who have written about the cases that stood out – troublemakers, alcoholics, abusers, gamblers, fighters, victims of accidents, and so on – and not about the majority of the thousands of *engagés* who were not, literally, remarkable. In other words, the exception has historically been considered the norm.

The figure I analyze in this article stands out because of his medical nature – voyageur Alexis Saint-Martin became an object of physiological experiment – an unusual occurrence in the voyageurs' corpus that, is, nevertheless, not so surprising considering the very physicality of the voyageur's way of life. Voyageurs worked extremely hard, existing in a constant state of survival, subjected to various injuries, and constantly at risk of dying in any of the hundreds of rapids they'd encounter on their voyages. They were paid only to toil, and their bodies were their tools. The particularity of the case of Saint-Martin and his doctor William Beaumont is that while Beaumont's writings originated from a very singular situation, they still deprived Saint-Martin of his singularity. By writing about Saint-Martin's injured body, and his perceived idiosyncrasy, Beaumont created a typical voyageur character out of an extraordinary one. It is another of such instances where the exception has fed the norm and contributed to the enduring folkloric images we still entertain today when we consider the role of the voyageur in Quebec and in North American history.

The story is well known. In 1822, a voyageur hired by the American Fur Company named Alexis Bidaguin *dit* Saint-Martin, born in 1802 in Berthier, Lower Canada (now Berthierville, Quebec), was the victim of a tragic blunder that should have killed him but didn't, becoming, instead, a historical event. At Mackinac Island's general store, a rendezvous for fur traders at the junction of Lakes Superior, Huron, and Michigan, Saint-Martin sustained an accidental rifle discharge at point-blank range that punctured his abdomen. Dr. William Beaumont, assistant surgeon to the US Army garrison stationed at Fort Mackinac was immediately called to the scene, where he saved Saint-Martin's life. In the following months and years that Dr. Beaumont treated Alexis Saint-Martin, the doctor was able to observe as Saint-Martin's wound healed, but not entirely, forming, rather, a fistula on his abdomen that provided direct access to his stomach via his abdominal wall. Seizing on the opportunity of this unexpected turn of events, Beaumont turned Saint-Martin into his guinea pig and studied and experimented on him for a decade. Thanks to his studies on Saint-Martin, Beaumont gained lasting international recognition and posterity in the medical annals, with his discoveries published in 1833.

And yet, 200 years after his accident and more than 140 years after his death in 1880, Alexis Saint-Martin still hasn't received the recognition he deserves.

This article is the first step in my endeavour to remedy this situation and consists of an analysis of Saint-Martin's initial representation by Beaumont. The most interesting studies of their case address the ethical aspects of their relationship, one of toxic codependency (Selzer) in a typical master-servant model of "informal domestic servitude" in Antebellum America (Green 193). These ethical issues will be addressed in this article but indirectly, as historical research can reveal the medical and cultural dimensions of hegemonic ideology in which the characters of Saint-Martin in particular, and of the voyageurs in general, were created: the writings of Beaumont reveal on their own the clearly unethical nature of his human experiments and the violent opinion he held of his guinea pig. This is the first in-depth character study of Alexis

Saint-Martin – which still hasn't been done, either in literary studies or in history – consisting of an analysis and a close reading of archivistic, medical, journalistic, and literary texts.

Little is known about Saint-Martin, while writings about the surgeon and his great destiny abound. Beaumont's book, *Experiments and Observations on the Gastric Juice and the Physiology of Digestion*,[1] which proved the chemical process of digestion through the acidity of gastric juices, was a critical milestone in our understanding of the human digestive system. And indeed, for the son of a modest Connecticut farming family to be recognized in medical history as the "Father of Gastric Physiology" is an accomplishment emblematic of the stubborn self-made man entirely dedicated to the realization of his American Dream. Beaumont had everything of the talented and brilliant opportunist, the go-getter who takes advantage of every opportunity, and provides History (with a capital "H") with a reservoir of stories and anecdotes conducive to his elevation to the rank of American hero. And Beaumont has certainly left a deep mark on both medical and military history: a large number of books and scientific, biographical, and historical articles affirm his relevance as the "first great American medical scientist" (Horsman) or note his resourcefulness as a "backwoods physiologist" (Osler, *An Alabama Student*) on the frontier. Hospitals and university pavilions bear his name, as do high schools, a gastroenterology award, and a highway in his hometown of Lebanon, Connecticut.

But Beaumont would never have achieved his fame without both the voluntary and coerced participation of his guinea pig Alexis Saint-Martin, who has but marginal recognition for his contribution to the advancement of science. This is probably due in part to the nature of the portrait Beaumont rendered of him. Beaumont first wrote of Saint-Martin in journals detailing his medical activities, then in two articles, "A Case of Wounded Stomach" (1825) and "Further Experiments on the Case of Alexis San Martin, Who Was Wounded in the Stomach by a Load of Buckshot" (1826), in his book *Experiments and Observations*, in various legal documents, and in his abundant correspondence. Because of Beaumont's position of power in relation to Saint-Martin, his representation of Saint-Martin became the basis of all those that would follow; Beaumont's portrait was considered authoritative, definitive.

On the one hand, the story of Saint-Martin, including voyageurs, agricultural life in the St. Lawrence Valley, complex North American geopolitics, and francophones' mass exodus to New England, is emblematic of

1 Plattsburgh, F.P. Allen, 1833. From this point on, I will cite the 1959 facsimile reprint of Beaumont's book with the acronym EO.

the nineteenth-century French Canadian history, but on the other hand, his incomplete and caricatured portrayal clearly demonstrates the overall lack of knowledge of North America's French-speaking culture in American literature. All these basic archetypal traits that together shape the textural character of Alexis Saint-Martin exist throughout the various texts authored by people other than Beaumont about this episode of medical history, mainly as an adjuvant of his success, and therefore as a secondary character in Beaumont's life.

## The Scientist's Supposed Objective Gaze

Creating a textual character from his elevated vantage point of scientist provided Beaumont the *a priori* of truth. His first words about Saint-Martin, however, show the incomprehension and incommunicability that would mark their relations to the end: "Alex Samata" is inscribed in disproportionate letters at the beginning of his journal entry, a mistake renewed once more in the upper margin with "San Maten," later corrected with "St. Martin" ("Journal of Cases" 12). As proof of this enduring misunderstanding, Beaumont continued to call his test subject "San Martin" in November 1825, in his article "Further Experiments," three and a half years after their first meeting. From the outset, in the doctor's gaze, this man with a fleeting identity is not a person in his own right; Saint-Martin is, instead, an anonymous voyageur, wrongly named because of the linguistic and cultural barriers, which Beaumont's deafness – the doctor became hard of hearing as an adolescent – would not help to lift. Different languages, religions, and social classes separated the soldier and scientist with considerable responsibilities and an illiterate who would never have had held any interest without this gunshot. Beaumont being hard of hearing would have made their communication all the more difficult.

Beaumont's journal entries on Saint-Martin are reproduced with the same wording in the *Medical Recorder* article of January 1825 (written in September 1824), in which Beaumont explains the care given to Saint-Martin to save his life and then facilitate the slow healing of the wound and its resorption into a fistula. This initial article would be used in *Experiments and Observations* as an introduction, augmented with the evolution of the case until the publication in 1833. The first four experiments carried out on Saint-Martin before his escape in 1825 were published in the second *Medical Recorder* article in 1826 and repeated in the same terms in the book. Since all these develop the same textual material, I will only observe the representation of Saint-Martin in the book, with which, with a rigorous scientific spirit and a probably accidental irony, Beaumont intends to submit "a body of facts" to the world (*Experiments and Observations* 6).

The poetics of this double meaning is enlightening. Saint-Martin, in Beaumont's book, is not considered in his entire complexity, but metonymized, reduced to a single part of his body, a wounded organ. Few details about Saint-Martin as an individual are revealed and often only indirectly. We must infer who Saint-Martin may have been and how he may have felt or how he may have behaved during those years of invasive experiments. Here is his first appearance:

> Alexis St. Martin, who is the subject of these experiments, was a Canadian, of French descent, at the above-mentioned time [1822] about eighteen years of age, of good constitution, robust and healthy. He had been engaged in the service of the American Fur Company, as a voyageur, and was accidentally wounded by the discharge of a musket, on the 6th of June, 1822. (9)

After this introductory paragraph, Saint-Martin's identity became optional and was most often ignored: his name only returns on page 18, and then from page 131, at the beginning of the second round of experiments in Prairie du Chien, Wisconsin, in 1829, when Saint-Martin and his young family joined Beaumont. Elsewhere, he is only a "youth" (9), a "man" (18, 20), or a "lad" (125), and he is mainly referred to by pronouns ("he," "him," "his"). His individuality fades behind the physiological phenomena that occur on and in his body, described objectively and in general terms as if it was not that of a full-fledged individual: "The projecting portion of the stomach was nearly as large as that of the lung" (10); "In five or six days there came away a cartilage, one inch in length" (15), and so on. We understand the erasure of the subject in such an experimental context; Beaumont doesn't intend to study the impact of emotions and behaviours on digestion, although, as we will see, emotions and behaviours inevitably influence it. This erasure is not only due to the objective rhetoric of scientific analysis. It is the first step in distancing Saint-Martin from himself, first reduced to a study subject,[2] then degraded, animalized, infantilized, and insulted throughout his correspondence.

2 "I gave him up as a lost subject for physiological experiment" (18), Beaumont said after Saint-Martin's first flight from Plattsburgh in 1825, where he accompanied Beaumont during a leave.

Still, Beaumont, in this introduction, doesn't hesitate to outline those aspects of his patient that shape his own figure as a scientist, affirming their relationship of subordination. Beaumont emphasizes the health and robust constitution of Saint-Martin and not for descriptive reasons. Beaumont's success at helping him to regain his strength, despite an injury that should have been fatal, proves his greatness as a doctor. He insists almost obsessively on this recovery: "From the month of April, 1823, at which time he had so far recovered as to be able to walk about and do light work, enjoying his usual good appetite and digestion, he continued with me, rapidly regaining his health and strength" (16); "In the spring of 1824 he had perfectly recovered his natural health and strength" (17); and again,[3] to the point of concluding his presentation by insisting on his vigour, which then seemed superior to that which he enjoyed before the accident: "Such has been this man's condition and circumstances for several years past; and now he enjoys the most perfect health and constitutional soundness, with every function of the system in full force and vigour" (20). Perhaps he does so to clear himself for having subjected Saint-Martin to experiments from which he coldly reveals the disabling effects in the rest of his book. The experiments' psychological effects, never taken into account in Beaumont's analyses or, for that matter, in their relationship, only filter in his book and correspondence.

Despite himself, Beaumont fleshes out Saint-Martin's character by giving him some of the classic attributes of the voyageur figure. Of course, Saint-Martin's strength and endurance were not due to his physician's surgical prowess, merited of their own accord. Both were necessary to his work, and to survive this accident, not to mention to sustain the exhaustive, painful operations that followed, and then to resume work as a voyageur, as he did during the first years he fled Beaumont, between 1825 and 1829: "he engaged with the Hudson Bay Fur Company, as a voyageur to the Indian country. He went out in 1827 and returned in 1828; and subsequently laboured hard to support his family" (18). Two more years as a lard eater (a *mangeur de lard*), doing a job that is difficult to conceive of today (sleeping in the bush, paddling, and portaging eighteen hours a day to Fort William [now Thunder Bay] and back to Montreal), was already a considerable task for anyone who did not have a gastric fistula.

But Beaumont elevated Saint-Martin's accomplishments to the rank of a larger-than-life figure. After two years in Prairie du Chien,

3 "he enjoyed perfect health" (18), "his health was good" (19), "He has been active, athletic and vigorous; exercising, eating and drinking like other healthy and active people." (20)

Saint-Martin returned to Berthier with his wife – Marie Joly – pregnant with twins, and their three children. Beaumont

> gave him an outfit for himself, wife, and children. They started in an open canoe, via the Mississippi, passing by St Louis, Mo.; ascended the Ohio river; then crossed the state of Ohio, to the Lakes; and descended the Erie, Ontario, and the River St. Lawrence, to Montreal, where they arrived in June. (19)

Here we have the feat of a voyageur who brings his wife and children alone, by canoe, from the West of the Great Lakes to Montreal. (Just imagine the family portage to pass Niagara Falls.) Regardless of whether they may have benefited at some point from naval transportation on the American rivers and Great Lakes, the image portrayed by Beaumont is that they traveled by canoe from March to June (c.f. the painting *The Trapper and his Family* [1845] by Charles Deas), Saint-Martin thus demonstrating his regained exceptional strength and endurance.

Moreover, not only does he have such stunning vigour, but he is immune to illness. In 1832, "he was in a midst of the cholera epidemic, at the time it prevailed and passed through Canada, and withstood its ravages with impunity, while hundreds around him fell sacrifices to his fatal influence" (19–20). In fact, from his healing with Beaumont until the end of the experiments in 1834, Saint-Martin "suffered much less predisposition to disease than is common to men of his age and circumstances in life" (20). Power and endurance,[4] as well as ironclad health,[5] are traits of the voyageur character canonized by Grace Lee Nute in her seminal work in 1931.

So too is the free and insubmissive spirit[6] Beaumont attributed to Saint-Martin, which lived on in the collective imagination. During the eleven years they intermittently worked together, Beaumont had

4 "[…] though the voyageur was short, he was strong. He could paddle fifteen – yes, if necessary, eighteen – hours per day for weeks on end and joke beside the campfire at the close of each day's toil. He could carry from 200 to 450 pounds of merchandise on his back over rocky portage trails at a pace which made unburdened travelers pant for breath in their endeavour not to be left behind." (Nute, 13)

5 "The men were not often sick […] Cox, an Astorian and a trader on the Pacific Coast, says of the men that they enjoyed good health and, with the exception of occasional attacks of rheumatism, were seldom afflicted with disease." (Nute, 91)

6 "[…] they were, nevertheless, very talkative, and independent in their way – Northwesters to the backbone […]"; "There is no life so happy as a voyageur's life; none so independent; no place where a man enjoys so much variety and freedom as in the Indian country," etc. (Nute, 206, 208)

control over his movements. He was in a position of authority over him, first for moral and caritative reasons after saving his life and taking him in his home in Mackinac,[7] then under contracts of engagement that Saint-Martin signed with an X in 1832 and 1833,[8] and finally as a military superior when Beaumont enlisted Saint-Martin in the American army to have him under his command and to pay for the institution. He had the good grace to allow him to return when the Black Hawk War in Michigan solicited him entirely as a military surgeon,[9] or when Alexis's father and eldest daughter died of cholera in 1832; otherwise, Beaumont kept him in his service "as a common servant" (19) and brought him with him on his many trips to New England. Saint-Martin's first escape in 1825, and his last in 1834, are considered by Beaumont as desertions: "From that latter place [Plattsburgh], he returned to Canada, his native place, without obtaining my consent" (18). In his second *Medical Recorder* containing the initial version of this excerpt, Beaumont had attributed a criminal character to Saint-Martin's flight: "The man absconded to Canada" ("Further Experiments" 97). These escapes nurture the myth of a selfish and disloyal Saint Martin, incapable of gratitude towards his saviour and benefactor.

Beaumont found nothing to reproach himself about, neither did his contemporaries nor his first commentators. In the letter he sent to James Webster, the publisher of the *Medical Recorder*, to introduce his second article, he regrets the ingratitude of Saint-Martin, who left despite the fact he was not suffering from the experiments: he was "unwilling to be experimented upon, though it caused him little pain or distress" (Myer 122). However, the manipulations, the very conditions in which the experiments took place, and their results prove Saint-Martin was suffering. For example, the "Mode of extracting the Gastric Juice" (21) by which Beaumont collected litres and litres of gastric juice over the years to use in his *in vitro* experiments and distributed liberally to chemists in the United States – and even in Sweden, where he sent a pint – involved inserting a rubber tube through the fistula into the empty stomach, irritating the membrane to secrete gastric juice, and moving it around to accentuate the secretion. "Its extraction is generally attended by that peculiar sensation at the pit of the stomach, termed sinking, with some

7 "He now entered my service." (EO, 19)

8 "In November 1832, he again engaged himself to me for twelve months, for the express purpose of submitting to another series of experiments." (EO, 20)

9 "In the spring of 1831, circumstances made it expedient for him to return with his family from Prairie du Chien to Lower Canada again. I relinquished his engagement to me for the time, on a promise that he would return when required…" (EO, 19)

degree of faintness, which renders it necessary to stop the operation," he notes (21). Other experiments consisted of suspending in the stomach any type of food attached by a string, or a bag of muslin containing the food, and removing them to see the state of digestion of the food after any given time. The movement of muslin bags in the stomach also caused this feeling of "pain and distress at the pit of the stomach" (251). Taking the internal temperature daily by inserting a thermometer into the orifice also leads to pain and dizziness. The practice revealed *in vivo* for the first time the movement of the sphincter of the pylorus, a muscle that regulates, through its contraction and expansion, the passage of the contents of the stomach into the duodenum; however, this movement, similar to deglutition, sought to swallow the thermometer in the body: "It would be drawn down towards the pyloric end, its whole length, ten or eleven inches, occasioning considerable distress, vertigo, and a sense of sinking at the *scrobiculus cordis*" (216). Whatever Beaumont told the publisher of the *Medical Recorder*, the first round of experiments, in August and September 1825, proved their severe inconvenience. These four experiments reveal both the suffering of the guinea pig and the slightly sadistic stubbornness of the researcher. The first deserves to be quoted extensively to illustrate what Saint-Martin had to submit to, infantilized as he was ("the lad," "the boy"), subordinated to the paternalism of his surgeon:

> At 2 o'clock, P.M., examined again – found the *a la mode beef* partly digested: the *raw beef* was slightly macerated on the surface, but its general texture was firm and entire. The smell and taste of the fluids of the stomach were slightly rancid; and the boy complained of some pain and uneasiness at the breast. Returned them again.
>
> The lad complaining of considerable distress and uneasiness at the stomach, general debility and lassitude, with some pain in his head, I withdrew the string, and found the remaining portions of the aliment nearly in the same condition as when last examined, the fluid more rancid and sharp. The boy still complaining, I did not return there anymore.
>
> *August* 2. The distress at the stomach and pain in the head continuing, accompanied with costiveness, a depressed pulse, dry skin, coated tongue, and numerous white spots, or pustules, resembling coagulated lymph, spread over the inner surface of the stomach, I thought advisable to give medicine; and, accordingly, dropped in the stomach, through the aperture, half a dozen *calomel pills*, four or five grains each .... (126)

Beyond this duly documented physical suffering, Saint-Martin was also subject to considerable psychological suffering, shown indirectly in Beaumont's analyses. During the above-mentioned experiment, the fact that Beaumont continued his manipulations in spite of Saint-Martin's pain ("Returned them again") shows the little consideration Beaumont accorded him, and indeed, Saint-Martin was not insensitive to these treatments, as evidenced by Beaumont's analysis of the effects of fear and anger on the state[10] of the stomach and its functioning.[11] While Beaumont cannot be accused of having maliciously provoked these psychological states (although fasting and physical activity were imposed regardless of their consequences[12]), there is no evidence that he sought to prevent them (he even indulged himself with veiled judgments regarding Saint-Martin's attitude[13]), and it's clear they proved very useful opportunities for study.

Moreover, Saint-Martin's suffering may have been indirectly expressed by the condition of his alcoholism. Obviously, it's impossible to isolate the causes of Saint-Martin's alcohol dependence, but one can intuit that post-traumatic shock caused by his injury; the humiliation of being paraded as a freak; the challenges of his infirmity; the chronic physical pain; the constant, invasive experiments; the exile from his country, his language, and his culture; and his separation from his family may surely have contributed to his illness. Here again, the problem of Saint-Martin's alcoholism has its merits, because it provides the opportunity for Beaumont to study the effect of alcohol on the state and functioning of the stomach ("the use of *ardent spirits always* produces disease of the stomach,"[14] he includes as the 13th of 51

---

10 "Derangement of the digestive organs, slight febrile excitement, fright, or any sudden affection of the passions, cause material alterations in his appearance. […] Fear and anger check its secretion, also: – the latter causes an influx of bile into the stomach, which impairs its solvent properties." (86–87)

11 For example, after the collection of bile contaminated gastric juice, Beaumont writes: "And this I suppose to have been the effect of violent anger, which occurred about the time of taking out this parcel. This experiment shows the effect of violent passion on the digestive apparatus. The presence of bile, in this instance, was believed to be the effect of anger." (153–154). After another experiment, he concludes that strong emotions slow digestion: "Another circumstance or two, may also, have contributed to interrupt the process of digestion, such as anger and impatience, which were manifested by the subject, during this experiment." (155)

12 "After breakfast, he exercised moderately. About 12 o'clock, M., he walked about two miles very quick. After his return to his lodging, he threw off his coat, and went in the open air again [on December 13th, 1832, in Washington, D.C.]. Soon after which, he began to feel the pain in his head, &c." (175)

13 "Feelings of impatience here evidently accelerated his pulse, in the erect position. He was vexed at being detained a few minutes from his breakfast." (184)

14 276. Beaumont emphasizes.

"Inferences" at the conclusion of his book). If Saint-Martin's alcoholism is addressed in the book, it is only for descriptive and analytical reasons: "appears to have been drinking liquor too freely" (236); "St. Martin has been drinking ardent spirits, pretty freely, for eight or ten days past" (237); "The free use of ardent spirits, wine, beer, or any intoxicating liquors, when continued for some days, has invariably produced these morbid changes [the diseased conditions of the coats of the stomach]" (239). Saint-Martin's drinking is judged negatively in Beaumont's correspondence and in the accompanying prefaces and concluding remarks of reissues of *Experiments and Observations.* This allows Beaumont, his interlocutors, and the book's prefacers to give to the character of Saint-Martin another characteristic trait of voyageur, one less glorious than superhuman strength or independence of mind: heavy drinking. As long as Beaumont sought to regain possession of him after his return home, Saint-Martin's alcoholism was a major problem. Beaumont and his emissaries were reluctant to advance money to finance Saint-Martin's return to the United States for fear that Saint-Martin would squander it. Clément Beaulieu, an agent of the American Fur Company near Trois-Rivières, wrote to Ramsay Crooks, then president of the company and a friend of Beaumont's:

> my opinion Sir it is a great risk to give St. Martin $100 in his hand in Canada first thing they will do when they get the money, is to close himself and his family and as he is a Drunkard he may spend the rest before he starts from this place, and then remain again as he did before. (Janowitz, 829–30)

Ramsay Crooks confirmed to Beaumont that Saint-Martin "had become such an abandoned drunkard" (Myer 83), and mentioned to William Morrison, another recruiting agent in Berthier that he was thus "utterly worthless" (Janowitz 831). Despite a period of moderate consumption in the 1840s, for which Beaumont personally congratulated him in a letter,[15] Saint-Martin' struggled with alcoholism until his death in 1880. His alcoholism was emphasized by the physician William Osler in an address in memory of Beaumont first published in 1902, then used as a preface to reissues of *Experiments and Observations* throughout the twentieth century. Osler quotes a judge from Berthier named Baby, who says of Saint-Martin: "When I came across him, he was rather poor, living on a small, scanty farm in St. Thomas, and very much addicted to drink, almost a drunkard

15 "I am happy to hear of your faithfulness & fidelity [as respects?] your engagements to me, as well as of the moral improvements of your life and habits. Continue to do so and & you will be duly rewarded by God and men." (March 28, 1846)

one might say" (*Experiments and Observations* xvii). The 1838 reissue included Scottish publisher Andrew Combe's thoughts that Beaumont's conclusions "confirmed [his] belief in the extent of mischief arising from [dietetic error], particularly in young men exposed to the temptation of drinking" (314–15), a general observation on the effects of consumption. But the inclusion of Osler's text in the preface to Beaumont's work then personalized this weakness in the face of temptation and contributed to the construction of Saint-Martin as an alcoholic character.

It's interesting to note that Beaumont didn't record Saint-Martin's alcohol consumption until the fourth and final round of experiments in Plattsburgh in 1833, so after ten years of collaboration. This doesn't mean, of course, that Saint-Martin didn't drink before this time. But it does suggest that Saint-Martin's consumption became such that, from this point on, it began to influence both the experiments and their results alike. No matter the consequences of Saint-Martin's living conditions with Beaumont, Saint-Martin's pain, or melancholy; no matter whether the twins his wife was pregnant with when they returned from Prairie du Chien in 1831 died in 1833 and 1834 or whether he lived in a state of constant mourning given the exceptionally high mortality rate in his family; no matter the psychological suffering caused by poverty, the influence of Saint-Martin's environment was never taken into consideration when judging his alcoholism. Subsequent literature considered that this flaw could only be a voyageur's atavism, therefore that of an irresponsible man, and the apostles of temperance in Lower Canada took Saint-Martin as a counter-example.

Together, these elements reveal the contradictions at work in Beaumont's creation of the textual character of Saint-Martin in his book. The author intends to offer science "a body of facts" by depersonalizing his subject of study and focusing on his stomach as if the organ were not attached to an individual, but he actually reveals Saint-Martin as a person, very well present in all the pages of the book, through the smallest secrets of his anatomy. It cannot be ignored that this is the description of the organ belonging to a man subjected to all these manipulations: a strong, resistant, stubborn, dissolute individual (in accordance with the myth of the voyageurs), who was also a sensitive, vulnerable, family-loving man who suffered physically and psychologically from his condition, from what was done to him, from what he was made to do.

## Beaumont's Subjectivity Takes Over

As discussed earlier regarding Saint-Martin's alcoholism, Beaumont's other writings, in dialogue with his immediate interlocutors, distort Saint-Martin's portrait. Without the filter of the scientific researcher's alleged objectivity, these writings modulate some of those characteristics already established in Beaumont's publications, but from the moment Saint-Martin severed his agreement with Beaumont, they mostly reveal the contempt and hatred the doctor has for his test subject. Saint-Martin's character becomes vile, cowardly, greedy, and despicable.

One of these documents is Beaumont's 1834 request for funding addressed to the American Congress in which he asks to be reimbursed for the cost of Saint-Martin's presence in his life. Given the objectives of his request (funding) and the people to whom it was addressed (members of Congress and not scientists), he darkened Saint-Martin's portrait to serve his needs:

> Alexis St. Martin, the person referred to, was an indigent inhabitant of the county of Michillimackinac, Mich. Ter. – not a soldier, but dependent entirely on his daily labor for his subsistence and support, and without friend or relative to take care of or provide for him in the misfortune which befell him. ("To the Honorable" 216)

Saint-Martin was no longer an American Fur Company *engagé* living on his wages, but a miserable inhabitant of the place, without family, colleagues, or a support system. Yet voyageurs formed a vibrant community with its own hierarchical structures, language, culture, and customs. Certainly, like his voyageur colleagues at the bottom of the ladder, Saint-Martin was neither rich nor privileged. But Beaumont, to emphasize his own magnanimity, presented him in his memoir as even more destitute than he was before his accident.

Of course, events made Saint-Martin dependent on all the help he could muster; yet Mackinac's authorities decided, after a year, a disabled voyageur did not deserve such expense. They declared him a "common pauper" and sought to send him back to Lower Canada in the next canoe leaving Mackinac. Beaumont claimed to have done everything to prevent his departure and to have resolved the issue

> as the only way to rescue St. Martin from impending misery and death, and to arrest the process of transportation and prevent the consequent suffering, by taking him into his own family, where all the care and attention were bestowed that his condition required.
>
> St. Martin was at this moment, as before intimated, altogether helpless and suffering under the debilitating effects of his wound – naked and destitute of everything. ("To the Honorable" 212–13)

Again, Beaumont exaggerated and carefully omitted to mention that Saint-Martin was then living with a woman named Mary Lafleur (Numbers 115) who provided him with the necessary care. Saint-Martin's situation, while serious, was further clouded by the erasure of the community with which he could identify and on which he could rely in his distress, in this case that of the French Canadians and the French-speaking Métis who lived permanently in Mackinac.

The depreciation of Saint-Martin continues by omission. In his memoir, Beaumont did not, as he did in his book to extol his medical prowess, portray a strong and enduring man. He merely mentioned Saint-Martin's healing, while specifying that it hindered his ability to keep him in his service, as Saint-Martin no longer required care for his survival and was no more than an object of research. This explains why Beaumont claimed to have paid for Saint-Martin's return from Mackinac to Montreal in 1825, when the truth was that Saint-Martin had actually fled Plattsburgh, proof of his will and dignity. By adding this false trip to the abundantly detailed expenses to be reimbursed, Beaumont created further reasons to complain about Saint-Martin's ingratitude. No domestic tasks his servant accomplished for him over a dozen years – not to mention the servant work his wife performed during the two years they spent at Prairie du Chien – is considered in his calculations: Beaumont claimed he received "no other indemnification at present than the thanks of an indigent man for the preservation of his life" ("To the Honorable" 214). In Beaumont's memoir, Saint-Martin is thus shown to be not only even more destitute than he really was, but incapable of gratitude to his benefactor – although he respected the moral debt that united them by refusing to collaborate with any other scientist until Beaumont's death in 1853.

It's obvious that Beaumont's depersonalization and fragmentation of Saint-Martin, by which the researcher isolated and objectified Saint-Martin's stomach as though it did not belong to him, were not due only to a scientific posture. Beaumont truly regarded Saint-Martin as subhuman, an inferior who belonged to him and whom he had to repossess at all costs after his departure. Beaumont considered Saint-Martin's refusal to submit to more experiments a great injustice. As mentioned above, the first two rounds of experiments were carried out with Saint-Martin's verbal agreement, a function of the moral debt because Beaumont had saved his life and taken him into his home. The following experiments, on the other hand, were conducted under contracts signed by Saint-Martin with the X of the illiterate. The contracts stipulated that Saint-Martin would "serve, abide, and continue with the said William Beaumont, wherever he shall go or travel, or reside in any part of the world,"[16] and that

16 "Articles of agreement…", October 16th, 1832. In Myer, 147. A second contract in 1833 was formulated in the same terms, with the only differences being the duration of the commitment, for two years this time, and remuneration.

> the said Alexis, will at all times during said term, when thereto directed or required by said William, submit to, assist and promote by all means in his power such Physiological or Medical experiments ... and will obey, suffer, and comply with all reasonable and proper orders or experiments of the said William. ("Articles of Agreement" 147–48)

It didn't matter whether or not Saint-Martin understood such legal jargon in a foreign language. He was now an indentured servant who would "obey, suffer, and comply." But Beaumont further strengthened his authority over Saint-Martin by having him enlist in the US Army Orderlies Reserve for five years, starting in December 1832, to have him under his direct command. Saint-Martin no longer belonged to himself but to an individual, according to the men's private agreements, and also to the state as a military orderly.[17]

Once his guinea pig left, never to return, Beaumont finally began to enjoy the notoriety he'd gained from his book and was solicited by scientists from the United States and Europe. He never reconciled himself to the loss of his object of study, however, which provoked anger and frustration that, as his correspondence revealed, would remain until his death in 1853. Some of Beaumont's correspondents continued to metonymize Saint-Martin by reducing him to his organ,[18] or simply to a dead weight to be delivered by boat "the same as baggage."[19] For Beaumont, Alexis Saint-Martin, his wife, and their children were but animals. This could not be more clearly stated than when he wrote to William Morrison "to inquire about my special pet" (February 1842)[20] or to his Plattsburgh cousin Samuel Beaumont about Saint-Martin's refusal to come to the United States without his family: "I must have him dead or alive, with or without his live stock" (April 4, 1846). Throughout the rest of his life, Beaumont openly expressed his contempt for "that old fistulous Alexis" (October 20, 1852), that "rascally Frenchman" (Horsman 205), that "reckless reprobate – faithless & intractable" (January 31, 1850, to W.G. Edwards), an individual so shabby that one could only look down on him with disgust and such a

17 It's in this spirit of State ownership that a defender of Beaumont's in the American Congress, during the debate on his memoir of 1834, asserted in a petition signed by more than two hundred elected officials that without financial support, the occasion "would be lost to our country forever." (Edward Everett to Secretary Lewiss Cass, in Myer, 229)

18 He is, for example, a "Patent Digester" according to Hercules L. Dousman, an officer of the American Fur Company. (November 13, 1837, letter)

19 William Morrison to Ramsay Crooks, May 15, 1839. In Janowitz, 831.

20 All dates in parentheses refer to letters in the Beaumont Archives at the Bernard Becker Medical Library Archives. See *BBMLA* entries in Works Cited.

sense of superiority ("if you can endure the disagreeable condescension of seeing Alexis," he wrote to Morrison (Myer 236)). He is willing to let Saint-Martin sink into poverty so that he can get him back, as he writes to US Army Surgeon General Joseph Lovell:

> I have taken no notice of his communication, nor shall I make any demonstrations to get him again till I return in the fall (which I hope to be permitted to do without fail), by which time he will have spent all the money I advanced him to provide for his family for the year ensuing, become miserably poor and wretched, and be willing to recant his villainous obstinacy and ugliness, and then I shall be able to regain possession of him again. (July 31, 1834)

This contempt is also expressed by the repeated assertion that Saint-Martin acted solely with intention to extort Beaumont, driven by lies,[21] "enjoying the fruits of ingratitude and injustice."[22] Beaumont's monetary offers to attract him to the United States were only "a bribe for his cupidity" (to Samuel Beaumont, October 20, 1852).

This degradation of Saint-Martin operates a reversal of power in the relationship that unites them. Beaumont considered himself the victim of the vile, exaggerated demands and shenanigans of his test subject. "I have evaded his designs so far" (October 20, 1852), Beaumont boasted to his cousin Samuel Beaumont in his final letter about Saint-Martin. This rhetoric, which positions Beaumont as the victim, was already present in his memoir to the Congress ("Your memorialist has been at great pains and expenses in relation to the individual whose care affords the facilities alluded to"; "your memorialist had not only to be at the trouble and expense of frequently seeking him in Canada after an unexpected absence of several years, but was obliged to pay him high wages" ("To the Honorable" 212, 213)), and it can be found in the evaluation of his memoir by congressmen (Chairman Sewall regretted "Dr. Beaumont's sacrifices of time and money in the prosecution of these experiments" (Myer 216)) and in the reception of his book (the elected P.C. Fuller touted "the efforts and the sacrifices required to procure St. Martin" (Myer 206)). With his numerous interlocutors and in his regular pleads for Saint-Martin to return, Beaumont never ceased to emphasize the disappointment and prejudice he caused him. This victimized tone

21 In his July 31, 1834 letter to Lovell, Beaumont writes a short poem on the theme: "This's just a snatch of Monsieur's ways. /Thus, go's he on in tricks and lies, /And thinks to get well paid for it."

22 Thus, Samuel Beaumont forwarded the words of his cousin to Saint-Martin in a letter on Jan. 12, 1835. In Myer, 235.

would be maintained from the first letter written to Surgeon General Joseph Lovell in 1834 after the definitive departure of Saint-Martin:

> A vexatious disappointment and an unexpected detention at Plattsburgh, awaiting Mons. Sergt. St. Martin's return to me at that place, prevented my arrival here several weeks sooner, and now I have the mortification to report him absent without leave. ... This placed me in a most unpleasant and vexatious predicament. (July 31, 1834)

to the last one he wrote in desperation to his guinea pig on October 15, 1852, addressed in French to *"Mon ami"*:

> Alexis, you know what I have done for you many years since; what I have been trying and am still anxious and wishing to do with and for you; what efforts, anxieties, anticipations, and disappointments I have suffered from your non fulfilment of my expectations. Don't disappoint me more, nor forfeit the bounties and blessings reserved for you. (October 15, 1852)

No wonder Beaumont saw himself as the aggrieved party in this relationship. Saint-Martin existed only to serve him, and so, outside the boundaries of this function, Saint-Martin did not, for all intents and purposes, exist: the overall animalization and fragmentation of Saint-Martin, the omissions, in Beaumont's memoir, of the communities to which Saint-Martin belonged when they collaborated (that of the voyageurs, that of the French Canadians and the French-speaking Métis of Mackinac and Prairie du Chien) and, when they no longer collaborated, Beaumont's intractable desire to prevent Saint-Martin from returning alongside his family. By isolating him and depriving him of what made him a relational subject belonging to collective and private spheres, by even denying his ability to feel pain, as one might with an animal, Beaumont deprived him of his humanity, of his identity: he was only a tool. In Beaumont's mind, he was himself the only party to encounter problems throughout his experiments and to have to overcome difficulties to accomplish his duties.

## The Caricature Casts a Long Shadow

William Beaumont, in the position of authority conferred to him by his status as surgeon, patron, and military superior, thus painted a unidirectional portrait of Alexis Saint-Martin. Under his pen, Saint-Martin began as a rich and contradictory character, at once astonishingly strong, tough, immune to disease, and a heavy drinker – all characteristics stemming from the myth of the voyageur – and also sensitive, fragile, loving his family, affected by deep physical and moral suffering. These last features, revealing the complexity of Saint-Martin's human condition, were subsequently excised from Saint-Martin in Beaumont's legal texts and correspondence, which gave way to his hatred and contempt for him. Saint-Martin was then depicted as an irresponsible, greedy, devious, ugly, vile, obstinate, and despicable character.

Thus, Beaumont's depiction of Saint-Martin in his non-scientific writings was much harsher than in his articles and book. Beaumont and his interlocutors found no positive traits in Saint-Martin, neither in his own person, nor in what actions he took, nor even in those he *did not take* by allowing himself to be studied so intrusively over the course of "his passive contribution to science," as wrote Jesse S. Myer, one of Beaumont's apologist biographers in 1912 (117). All human beings have their weaknesses and flaws, and Saint-Martin certainly had no shortage of them. Beaumont's caricatured portrait of his test subject, however, lacks the humanity or even the slightest empathy that would have made it possible to portray their relationship as what it really was, one of co-dependence.

If the obvious ethical questions raised by their relationship weren't touched on in this essay, it's because Beaumont himself didn't consider them, and therefore the studied corpus did not immediately address them. In fact, Beaumont's contemporaries reproached him only for not having tried harder to close Saint-Martin's wound right from the start, and never questioned the nature of his experiments, or of their specifically medically indentured relationship. Neither the medical practices nor the times allowed for such critical self-evaluation, and this negative portrait of Saint-Martin, created by a man whose judgment was never doubted, remained authoritative for over a century. For example, here is what physiologist Arno Luckhardt said in 1939 about a letter written in Saint-Martin's name and preserved in Beaumont's archives at the University of Chicago:

> Facsimile of a letter by Alexis St. Martin written and addressed to Dr. Beaumont for the illiterate St. Martin by some unknown Canadian amanuensis (probably the parish priest). The translated text of this letter representative of many others written by the surly, irresponsible, pecunious, ungrateful ward and human guinea pig to his solicitous, merciful, and generous benefactor reads as follow. (Luckhardt 551)

The lasting contempt that Saint-Martin has inspired could hardly be more explicit. It wasn't until the 1950s, after the Nuremburg trials, that historians and the medical community began to question the ethics of Beaumont's experiments and tried to nuance the unilateral portrait Beaumont had made of Saint-Martin. One of the first to do so was

Edward Bensley, a member of a committee appointed by the Physiological Society of Canada for the recognition of Saint-Martin in the medical history, and Dr. Sylvio Leblond in the 1960s, one of the few Quebecers to be interested in Saint-Martin.

Saint-Martin's figure and personal history still have yet to be completely understood or appropriately contextualized. In literature, the latest novel on Beaumont's life, *Open Wound*, by the American surgeon Jason Karlawish (2011), does attempt to grant Saint-Martin some subjectivity through individual traits – like a talent for wood carving – but Karlawish's lack of knowledge of French Canada lends his representation comically artificial tones, like when Saint-Martin speaks with Parisian expressions ("*Putain, ça craint!*"). In Quebec, only one novel features Saint-Martin as the protagonist (*Alexis Saint-Martin (1794* [sic]*–1880) L'homme-cobaye du Docteur William Beaumont*, Serge Gauthier, 2021), but Gauthier takes significant liberties with dates and facts – such as rendering Saint-Martin an avid reader and prolifically epistolical – and mines such voyageur tropes as superhuman strength, irresistible sexual charisma, or a talent for hunting so incredible that fur trading agents know who he is even before he arrives for his first engagement. Both novels rely on commonplace historical voyageur characteristics that still contribute to the superficial representation of the profession today.

My close analysis of the portrait of Saint-Martin made by Beaumont and others will contribute to better understanding who he was – not only as an actor in these critical scientific discoveries – but as a man of his day and age and condition, an individual who lived a rich life worthy of consideration far beyond its more sensational aspects. Furthermore, the study of Saint-Martin will contribute to the complexification of the French Canadian voyageur figure, which lacks both depth and realism. Saint-Martin's life is not just a story of abuse, and suffering, and systemic coercion, it is also one of family and community cohesiveness and the pursuit of dignity through an entire spectrum of emotions. The French-Canadian *voyageur* figure, in popular culture, has yet to embody the complexity of the human condition, and, through my work as a writer and researcher, I hope to help remedy these shortcomings, if only in part.

## WORKS CITED

Beaumont, William. "A Case of Wounded Stomach." *The Medical Recorder*, vol. 8, no. 1, Jan. 1825, pp. 14–19.

–. "Further Experiments on the Case of Alexis San Martin, Who Was Wounded in the Stomach by a Load of Buckshot." *The Medical Recorder*, vol. 9, no. 1, Jan. 1826, pp. 94–97.

–. *Experiments and Observations on the Gastric Juice and the Physiology of Digestion*. 1833. Dover Publications, 1959.

–. "*Articles of Agreement …*" Myer, pp. 147–49.

–. "*To the Honorable, The Senate and House of Representatives of the United States of America, in Congress Assembled*." Myer, pp. 212–15.

–. "Journal of Cases in W. Beaumont's Medical Practice, Including Earliest Descriptions of the Wounding of St. Martin, Recorded at Fort Mackinac, MI. 18 Nov. 1822–12 Jan. 1825." Washington U School of Medicine. *Bernard Becker Medical Library Archives*. http://digitalcommons.wustl.edu/beaumont_1812_1827/16. Accessed 24 June 2022. The Beaumont Archives will now be referred to by the acronym BBMLA.

– to Lovell, Joseph. 31 July 1834. *BBMLA*, http://digitalcommons.wustl.edu/beaumont_1834/17. Accessed 24 June 2022.

– to Morrison, William. Feb. 1842. *BBMLA*, http://digitalcommons.wustl.edu/beaumont_1842/10. Accessed 24 June 2022.

– to Beaumont, Samuel. 4 Apr. 1846. *BBMLA*, http://digitalcommons.wustl.edu/beaumont_1846/23. Accessed 24 June 2022.

– to Edwards, W.G. 31 Jan. 1850. *BBMLA*, http://digitalcommons.wustl.edu/beaumont_1849_1850/7. Accessed 24 June 2022.

– to Saint-Martin, Alexis. 15 Oct. 1852. *BBMLA*, http://digitalcommons.wustl.edu/beaumont_1851_1879/12. Accessed 24 June 2022.

– to Beaumont, Samuel. 20 Oct. 1852. *BBMLA*, http://digitalcommons.wustl.edu/beaumont_1851_1879/11. Accessed 24 June 2022.

Combe, Andrew. "Concluding Remarks by the Editor." *Experiments and Observations*, Beaumont, pp. 303-19.

Deas, Charles. *The Trapper and his Family*. 1845. *MFABoston*, https://collections.mfa.org/objects/269844.

Gauthier, Serge. *Alexis Saint-Martin (1794–1880): L'homme-cobaye du Docteur William Beaumont*. Éditions Charlevoix, 2021.

Green, Alexa. "Working Ethics. William Beaumont, Alexis St. Martin, and Medical Research in Antebellum America." *Bulletin of the History of Medicine*, vol. 84, no. 2, summer 2010, pp. 193–216. https://doi.org/10.1353/bhm.0.0341.

Horsman, Reginald. *Frontier Doctor: William Beaumont, America's First Great Medical Scientist*. U of Missouri P, 1996. Missouri Biography Series.

Janowitz, Henry D. "Newly Discovered Letters Concerning William Beaumont, Alexis Saint-Martin and the American Fur Company." *Bulletin of the History of Medicine*, vol. 22, no. 6, 1948, pp. 822–32.

Karlawish, Jason. *Open Wound: The Tragic Obsession of Dr. William Beaumont*. U of Michigan P, 2011.

Lavigne, Nicole. *L'étonnante destinée de Pierre Boucher*. Québec Amérique, 2021.

Luckhardt, Arno. "Medical History Collections in the United States and Canada. I. The Doctor Beaumont Collection of the University of Chicago." *Bulletin of the History of Medicine*, vol. 7, no. 5, 1939, pp. 535–63.

Myer, Jesse S. *William Beaumont, a Pioneer American Physiologist*. Mosby, 1981, 1912.

Numbers, Ronald L. "William Beaumont and the Ethics of Human Experimentation." *Journal of the History of Biology*, vol. 12, no. 1, 1979, pp. 113–35.

Nute, Grace Lee. *The Voyageur*. Minnesota Historical Society, 1931.

Osler, William. "William Beaumont, A Pioneer American Physiologist." *The Journal of the American Medical Association*, vol. 39, no. 20, 15 Nov. 1902, pp. 1223–31. https://doi.org/10.1001/jama.1902.52480460001001

–. *An Alabama Student and Other Biographical Essays*. Oxford UP, 1909.

–. "A Pioneer American Physiologist." Introduction. Beaumont, *Experiments and Observations*, 1959, pp. i–xix.

Paré, Étienne. "Nominations controversées au Prix France-Québec." *Le Devoir*, 30 April 2022. https://www.ledevoir.com/lire/705588/prix-litteraire-france-quebec-nominations-controversees-au-prix-france-quebec. Accessed 15 Dec. 2023.

Rainville, Raymond. *1542: La Colonie Maudite*. Éditions La Plume d'or, 2022.

Selzer, Richard. "Alexis St. Martin." *Confessions of a Knife*. Simon and Schuster, 1979, pp. 116–32.

# 3 The Material Turn of "Japs" in John Okada's *No-No Boy*[1]

CHANG-HEE KIM

## The Eugenic Blending of History, Ideology, and Memory in the United States

Eugenic knowledge operates as a biopolitical force that sustains social hierarchies by categorizing humans into binary groups based on abstract, biological, or material constructs of good versus evil, beauty versus ugliness, and differences in race, gender, sexuality, and other bodily traits. By exploiting physical variations in the human body, eugenic ideology justifies discriminatory practices and enforces notions of superiority at the population level. Historically, eugenic values tied to beauty and health have been projected onto white bodies, positioning them as benchmarks of societal normalcy. Whiteness, in particular, has been imbued with racial privilege and supremacy, underpinned by the baseless notion that dark skin is "unhealthy and unfit." These unfounded beliefs about dark skin lie "at the heart of scientific racism and eugenic ideologies and policies" (Benjamin 56). Furthermore, eugenic ideologies instil in Black people the belief that their bodies symbolize "ugliness, sin, darkness, and immorality," as Frantz Fanon observes (188). This internalization drives the perception that colonialism might redeem their perceived "darkness," creating a perpetual internal conflict as they remain "forever in combat with [their] own image" (189). This racialized psychological mechanism mirrors what Ngũgĩ wa Thiong'o terms "colonizing the mind." It reflects the disciplinary power of colonial ideology over the racial corporeality and identity of the colonized, fostering

1 This chapter is an expanded and revised version of my article, originally written in Korean and titled "The Cold War Biopolitics of Disability in John Okada's *No-No Boy*: Racialized and Gendered Ableism of American Society in the 1950s," which was published in the Korean journal *Modern Fiction in English* in 2022.

self-hatred and triggering a psychological process that leads to cultural erasure, de-historicization, and de-subjectification (72).

The biased perception of hygiene imposed on Black skin is rooted in eugenic principles embedded within the colonial bio-politics of a society shaped by white dominance. This prejudiced view, particularly prevalent in the United States, frames the racial materiality of people of colour as an external pathogen to be eliminated for societal security, thereby invalidating the legitimacy of Black racial identity. Moreover, discrimination based on physical differences fosters an ableist ideology, normalizing stigmatization and hostility towards those perceived as deviating from the norm. This perpetuates the ideal of able-bodiedness and expands the boundaries of what is considered pathologically disabled.

In *The Bluest Eye*, for example, Toni Morrison explores how Blackness, embodied in the Black body, becomes an emotionally and culturally charged concept of disability during the 1940s. This novel intricately examines the intersections of body, substance, and agency, contrasting the lived experiences of Blackness with the dominant white, middle-class American standard of beauty. As Naomi Rand describes, this standard represents "the power of white iconography" (59), shaping the narrative's discourse on the material and ideological implications of the Black body. Set in the late 1940s, the novel portrays a period when Blackness was systematically denied within the white supremacist framework of US bio-power. Pecola, the protagonist, is a figure marked by a constellation of socially denigrated traits: Black skin, female gender, poverty, incestuous pregnancy, and a family stigmatized as "ugly people" (39). These attributes position her in stark opposition to the normative ideal of the "perfect" American body. As a result, Pecola becomes a "desiring machine," yearning for whiteness – its flesh, its skin, and its symbolic power. Her desperate longing manifests in schizophrenic neurosis, reflecting what Malin W. Pereira describes as "a cultural insanity threatening the Black community's identity and strength" (74).

Pecola's disabled ontology underscores the pervasive racism of mid-twentieth-century white America. Yet, her Black body, as a desiring machine, undergoes constant transformation, emerging affectively as a (dis)abled subjectivity – a Black body with the bluest eyes. This transformation reveals the fraught intersections of race, beauty, and disability within an oppressive social framework. Pecola's existential crisis – caught between the longing for white acceptance and the societal rejection of Black identity – exposes the ideological mechanisms of white iconographic power.

Pecola's plight embodies an unreproducible madness rooted in the American ideal of the family during the late 1940s. However, as Carl

Malmgren notes, the blue-eyed Pecola is not solely her own; her essential materiality transcends individual existence (259). Pecola undergoes a profound ontological transformation, shifting from a black-skinned girl to one with the bluest eyes. Her blind yearning for whiteness leads her to lose her sanity, yet in this state, she is no longer governed by external forces. This aligns with Gilles Deleuze's concept of a "body without organs," where Pecola's vital materiality constitutes a complex multiplicity beyond herself, disrupting social norms and exposing sites of internal and external rupture. Echoing Deleuze and Guattari's concept of the "desiring machine," Pecola, as noted in *Dialogues II* (Deleuze and Parnet 89), is ultimately "deprived of the power of saying 'I.'"

Pecola's desire for blue eyes exemplifies how eugenic racism in America, shaped by the interaction of social, cultural, and psychological mechanisms surrounding the Black body, operates as a productive, transformative, yet pathological force, driven by her internalized deficiency or longing for whiteness. In fact, the history of racism in America reveals how such individual desires are cultivated within the social framework of US eugenics, which has shaped the intertwined relationship between race, genetics, and social inequality in the formation of public policies and societal norms. In 1924, for instance, the United States enacted a series of anti-immigration laws designed to restrict Asian immigration, reflecting the social evolutionary ideologies that would later influence Hitler's policies of Aryan racial superiority and culminate in the Holocaust. These laws coincided with the publication of Hitler's *Mein Kampf*. The origins of such exclusionary measures date back to the Chinese Exclusion Act of 1882, which marked a pivotal moment in US history, challenging the nation's self-image as a land of opportunity and freedom.

These policies sought to curtail the growth of Asian populations by banning interracial marriages and reducing immigration quotas. In a similar vein, historian Ann G. Winfield argues that US history is steeped in "base racism, ethnic hatred, and academic elitism," employing eugenic principles to counter what Theodore Roosevelt described as "racial suicide" and to promote Nordic superiority (xviii). Winfield further notes that US education has uniquely intertwined "history, ideology, and children" since its inception (xviii–xix). Roosevelt, an advocate of social evolutionism and the doctrine of Manifest Destiny, oversaw the annexation of the Philippines, a move justified by Rudyard Kipling's depiction of colonized peoples as "half devil and half child" in his poem "The White Man's Burden." Kipling framed it as the United States' duty to assimilate the "new-caught, sullen peoples" into the expanding empire, compelling them to "go to school for better or worse" as part of a paternalistic mission to civilize (Dalrymple 64; Zimmerman 28).

The distinctive interplay of history, ideology, and memory – intricately weaving material connections between actors and space-time – holds the potential to mitigate the destructive impulses of assembled forces. The prevailing social order endeavours to achieve a normative organic unity amid inherent differences. However, maintaining this order requires the containment of heterogeneous actors and actants, whose latent capacities for disruption challenge the status quo.[2] Gilles Deleuze and Félix Guattari's concept of assemblage, defined within the collective expanse of plateaus and described as a "plane of consistency" (*A Thousand Plateaus* 4), illustrates this containment.[3] Yet, within the interconnected fabric of reality, discriminatory systems such as racism, sexism, classism, and ableism function as loci of social resistance or justice, where the rhizomatic movements of actors and actants subvert containment and repression. These dynamics transform assemblages into fertile grounds for reconfiguration. Consequently, the governance of existing hierarchies may collapse, transform, and reassemble, continually generating new relations between human and non-human actors and actants and (de)constructing desires, materials, and boundaries (Deleuze and Parnet 69).[4]

---

2 In literary and cultural theory, the term *actor* generally refers to someone or something performing actions within a narrative, often associated with specific identities who have personal traits, motivations, and developments. In comparison, *actant*, a concept from structural semiotics, denotes functional roles within a narrative, focusing on the functions or roles participants fulfil rather than their specific identities in the structure of the narrative.

3 Deleuze and Guattari's concept of assemblage refers to a dynamic, complex configuration of heterogeneous elements that come together to form a temporary and contingent unity. This framework highlights the fluid, interconnected nature of these components, rejecting rigid hierarchies and fixed structures. In *A Thousand Plateaus*, they argue that reality is composed of these assemblages, which can include both human and non-human elements. The idea of assemblage aligns with their broader philosophical concepts, including their critique of essentialism, emphasis on becoming and process, and exploration of non-hierarchical, rhizomatic structures.

4 Scholars in Asian American studies engage with continental philosophy, including the ideas of Deleuze and Guattari, in diverse and varied ways, resulting in a non-uniform reception of these ideas within the field. For instance, Min Hyoung Song finds Deleuze and Guattari's rhizomatic thinking valuable for challenging linear and essentialist narratives about Asian American experiences. The concept of rhizomes, which resists hierarchical structures, can be used to understand the complexity and interconnectedness of Asian American identities. In this sense, continental philosophy, particularly post-structuralist thought, provides tools for deconstructing essentialist notions of identity in Asian American studies, allowing for a deeper analysis

However, the struggle among particles in the assemblage does not follow a linear, binary, or easily cross-sectional path. Like the agential subject of the desiring machine, it emerges as a dynamic force in perpetual flux, dismantling established structures while forging new connections. Yet these movements are diverse, lacking coherence or dialectical patterns, and often operate through complex causality. This complexity can lead to unintended consequences, including reinforcing or exacerbating existing forms of discrimination. For instance, the American Blind Veterans Association rejected hierarchies based on physical differences such as disability, only to uphold hierarchies rooted in race. This undermines the moral coherence of resistance movements and erodes their ideological foundation (Nielsen 156).

This chapter deals with the embodied experiences of Japanese Americans assimilating into the post-war US assemblage of the 1950s, focusing on their dual marginalization as both ontologically negated and corporeally excluded from the normative framework of what it meant to be American. Using John Okada's 1957 novel *No-No Boy* as a critical lens, the analysis explores how Japanese Americans – interned during World War II and subsequently reintegrated – navigated the complex sociopolitical landscape of post-war American life. The novel portrays characters grappling with alienation, despair, anxiety, madness, and hope within a society defined by containment and integration. Okada's work parallels Joy Kogawa's 1981 novel *Obasan*, which reflects on the internment experiences of individuals of Japanese descent in Canada during and after World War II. Both texts underscore the dislocation, adversity, and community breakdown wrought by internment, prompting psychoanalytic interpretations that address the collective trauma of its aftermath. Critics such as Jinqui Ling, Viet Nguyen, and Daniel Y. Kim recognize *No-No Boy* as a critical text that captures the post-war atmosphere in 1940s and 1950s America. During this period, Japanese Americans often felt compelled to sever "all traces and ties" to their ethnic identity to avoid discrimination (Abe and Imamura 274).

---

of how categories like *Asian American* are constructed, contested, and decentered. On the other hand, scholars such as Lisa Lowe critique continental philosophy for being Eurocentric and insufficiently attentive to the specificities of Asian American experiences. They argue that it may not fully capture the nuances of racialized experiences within the Asian American context. Despite these critiques, many scholars in the field engage with continental philosophy in a critical and transformative manner, drawing on key concepts while simultaneously challenging and expanding theoretical frameworks to better address the unique aspects of Asian American experiences. For more details, see Song's chapter "Desert-Orient-Nomad" in *The Children of 1965: On Writing, and Not Writing*.

The 1950s US context, described by Daniel Kim as an "empire of feeling" (77), was marked by dual narratives of containment and integration.[5] This era juxtaposed the looming threat of nuclear war with an emphasis on family values and the fragile coexistence of segregation and liberalism. Amid Cold War tensions, the American home was idealized as a "bastion of [a] home-front defense, fighting unit" (Jonnes 29) and a "bulwark against the dangers of the Cold War" (May xviii). This ethos rationalized the American way of life, casting people of colour, women, the disabled, and other marginalized groups as abnormal or deviant. Japanese Americans, under this pressure, were compelled to adopt an American identity, suppressing their inherent ethnic materiality. In *No-No Boy*, this shift is evident as Japanese Americans navigate integration and survival, striving to "blend into mainstream American society" (Ng 103) within the Cold War framework.

That said, this chapter examines Okada's novel to explore how the assemblage of history, ideology, and memory shaped the productive, transformative, and pathological desires invoked by American eugenics during World War II. Adopting a materialist approach to Okada's ableist narrative, the chapter interrogates how it displaces the illegitimate materiality of those labelled as "no-no boys" or "Japs" – a complex identity that transcends both Japanese and American origins. Through this lens, the analysis traces how the Japanese American body internalizes and appropriates the eugenic ideology of ableism prevalent at the time in its quest for a "point of wholeness and belonging" (Okada 138). Ultimately, this chapter reveals how this process reflects a distinctive interplay of history, ideology, and memory within the socio-political fabric of 1950s America.

## Negation and Negativity in No-No Boys' Bodies

Following the 1941 attack on Pearl Harbor, President Franklin D. Roosevelt issued Executive Order 9066, mandating the forced removal and

5 The concept of the "empire of feeling" (D. Kim 77) highlights the pervasive influence of emotional and affective dimensions in shaping social and political structures within specific historical and cultural contexts. It refers to the collective emotional atmosphere or prevailing sentiments of a society or era that significantly influence individual and collective behaviours, attitudes, and responses. In the context of Okada's *No-No Boy* and postwar America, the empire of feeling encompasses the dominant emotions and sentiments – fear, prejudice, loyalty, and patriotism – that shaped the complex socio-political landscape. This emotional terrain, shaped by factors such as the aftermath of World War II, the Cold War, racial tensions, and the treatment of Japanese Americans, particularly those ostracized for their wartime decisions regarding loyalty, reveals the profound interplay between emotion and societal structures.

incarceration of Japanese nationals and Americans of Japanese descent from the western mainland and Hawaii. These individuals were relocated to makeshift internment camps in remote inland desert areas, including Nevada and Arizona. Their properties were confiscated or sold at drastically reduced prices to white neighbours, as "no one wanted to buy things from Japan" (Ng 102). This act reduced Japanese Americans to what Giorgio Agamben terms "bare life," stripping them of the rights and protections that constitute "political life." In 1948, Congress passed a bill aimed at compensating those affected by the executive order. However, addressing the profound trauma of being treated as enemies by their own country proved far more challenging, and the economic losses remained largely unresolved (Ng 102). This enduring legacy is poignantly reflected in Mike Shinoda's 2005 song "Kenji," which recounts his father's internment experiences. Through his lyrics, Shinoda expresses the generational psychological scars and the persistent stigma encapsulated by the refrain, "Japs not welcome anymore!" (Shinoda).

Amid this historical backdrop, John Okada published *No-No Boy* during an era when Japanese Americans were "busy keeping their heads down, assimilating, and working on becoming a model minority of 1950s America" (Ozeki viii). The novel delves into the aftermath of Japanese-American internment during World War II, set against the post-war landscape of Seattle. It examines themes of loyalty, discrimination, and the struggle for self-acceptance in a nation reckoning with its wartime actions and prejudices. The protagonist, Ichiro Yamada, is a "no-no boy," having answered negatively to two controversial loyalty questions posed by the government: whether he would serve in the US military and whether he would forswear allegiance to Japan. His refusal resulted in a two-year prison sentence. The novel chronicles Ichiro's internal conflicts over identity and belonging, as well as the broader societal struggles faced by Japanese Americans as they attempted to reintegrate into civilian life following their internment. Through its deeply personal narrative, *No-No Boy* offers a powerful exploration of the lasting impacts of war, prejudice, and displacement.

The novel opens with Ichiro returning to his hometown of Seattle after two years of incarceration. Through an omniscient narrative, Okada portrays Ichiro as an "intruder" in his own community (Okada 3). Japanese Americans, often labelled as "perpetual foreigners," shared certain experiences with other Asian immigrants in America. However, unlike other immigrants, Japanese Americans had no homeland to return to – their homes had been confiscated, and their sovereign rights revoked. Upon his return, Ichiro encounters hostility from his old friend Eto, who, upon learning that Ichiro is a no-no boy, derisively calls him a traitor (5). This sets the stage for a central question in the novel: how can Ichiro, stripped of his birthright and sovereign rights, reclaim legitimacy and belonging in post-war America? Moreover, how might his "un-American" body be reconfigured within the sociopolitical fabric of what it meant to be American during that era?

Okada's narrative directly engages with the stigma faced by Japanese Americans, whose claim to an American identity was systematically denied. It seeks to address the psychological and physical wounds of those whose identities were fractured by wartime incarceration and its aftermath. The dual negative of "no-no" casts Japanese Americans as doubly negated – culturally, socially, and politically excluded from Americanness. Ichiro's own family serves as an example of this erasure. While Ichiro dutifully honours his parents' cherished Japanese heritage, he is branded a "rotten, no-good bastard" (5) by his peers and even his younger brother, Taro. Taro, rejecting the inherited materiality of Japanese identity within the family, grows resentful of his no-no boy brother. This resentment climaxes when Taro violently repudiates Ichiro by physically attacking him with friends and severing ties with his family to join the military, seeking to affirm his Americanness.

Isolated even within his own home, Ichiro embarks on a fraught journey to find his place in post-war American life. He grapples with conflicting emotions: resentment toward his parents for their role in shaping his identity, compassion for their struggles, and envy of "yes-yes boys" like his veteran friend, Kenji, who embody a more socially accepted model of Americanness. Okada's narrative critiques the incompatibility of Ichiro's "un-American" family with the dominant Cold War culture of containment, conformity, and family ideology that characterized 1950s America. Ultimately, the novel resolves the tension within Ichiro's family through the tragic suicide of his mother, Mrs. Yamada, and the symbolic emasculation of his father. These events underscore what Apollo Amoko identifies as the novel's "troubling disavowal of all traces of Japanese heritage" (47). By neutralizing the no-no boy family's dynamics, Okada's *No-No Boy* interrogates the costs of cultural assimilation and the fractured identities of Japanese Americans in the aftermath of war and internment.

In contrast to Ichiro, Kenji, a World War II veteran, embodies the normative ideal of an American, transcending even the expectations of the model minority despite his Japanese heritage. Benefiting from the government's G.I. Bill, Kenji's family enjoys a level of affluence that perfectly aligns with the 1950s myth of middle-class prosperity, complete with suburban housing, automobiles, children, and educational opportunities. This positive portrayal of the yes-yes boy's family starkly contrasts with the dysfunctionality of Ichiro's no-no boy family, which is marred by anger, guilt, insanity, violence, and death. Okada's narrative presents Ichiro's family as a hostile entity, fundamentally excluded from the 1950s American way of life. Their perceived "unhealthy and unfit" state of disability renders them inadequate according to societal norms, with their foundational ties to Japanese language, culture, and body symbolizing "all traces and ties" to Japanese heritage that must be eradicated. Kenji's family serves as the antithesis, highlighting the novel's embrace of "an assimilationist conception of citizenship, normative lifestyles, and the compulsory conformity to an abled body and mind" (Chen 28).

The novel further critiques the ableist yet guilt-ridden social ethos of the 1950s, epitomized by Mr. Carrick – a white man of "money and position and respectability" (Okada 135). Carrick's acknowledgement of the "mistake" committed against people of Japanese descent contributes to Ichiro's ontological transformation, as Carrick extends acceptance to Ichiro as an American. Characters like Mr. Carrick embody the politically correct liberal agenda of 1950s middlebrow culture, aligning with the broader Cold War narrative of the United States, which sought to "[win] the friendship of Asians" (Klein 88). Christina Klein identifies this as "Cold War Orientalism," a framework characterized by efforts at "global imaginary integration." These liberal attitudes, reminiscent of today's affirmative action, enable Ichiro to embark on a material turn, culminating in his realization: "It's a matter of attitude. Mine needs changing" (Okada 186).

In the following section, this chapter explores how no-no boys, whose identity is "ornamented" with the stigma of being "Japs" within the American way of life in the 1950s, undergo such a material turn. It examines the ways in which their ontological dislocation is reconfigured through societal forces, ultimately revealing the tensions between assimilation, identity, and the residual trauma of wartime incarceration.

## The Japanese Body, Disability, and Difference-in-Itself

As Kim Nielsen asserts, US society has historically associated disability with specific groups based on race, gender, class, and sexuality, using it as a tool to justify systemic discrimination. In the case of Asian migrants, Americans often perceived them as lacking "able-bodiedness," framing them as deficient in linguistic or intellectual capabilities (Nielsen 3). This perception extended to judgments of their intelligence, rendering their bodies "too disabled for democracy" (105). An in-depth examination of the interplay between history, ideology, and the memory of disability in 1950s America reveals a causal relationship between the racialized disabilities imposed on Japanese American bodies and their internalized aspiration for ableism, projected onto the idealized whiteness of the era.

In this context, Ruth Ozeki observes that Okada's *No-No Boy* resonated deeply with the Japanese body, metaphorically reopening old wounds, which may explain why the novel went out of print shortly after its initial release in the 1950s (viii). By contrast, Kogawa's *Obasan* addresses the lasting impact of internment camps on Japanese Canadians, including the mutilation of their bodies and the psychological scars caused by the atomic bombings in Japan. Kogawa's novel transcended literature, becoming a political force that galvanized societal awareness of historical injustices and wrongs committed by the Canadian government. Her work played a pivotal role in fostering a national consensus, culminating in a formal government apology.

Okada's novel, however, focuses on the psychological and physical struggles of Japanese Americans attempting to reintegrate into a post-war society rife with anti-Asian racism. Rather than driving political reform, *No-No Boy* explores the bio-political landscape where racial and gendered ableism impose insanity, hatred, stigma, and physical and metaphorical amputation on the "no-no" bodies of the "Japs." This bio-political lens underscores how these bodies are burdened with societal rejection, rendering their desperate efforts towards belonging and self-acceptance seemingly futile. Through this portrayal, Okada captures the deep fractures within a society grappling with its own contradictions in the wake of war and exclusion.

Ableism surfaces prominently in *No-No Boy* through the stark material and symbolic disparities in femininity between Mrs. Yamada and Emi, Ichiro's female friend. Mrs. Yamada embodies the antithesis of the gender expectations imposed by 1950s American family ideology, particularly those placed on women and wives. She assumes the de facto role of head of the household in place of her ineffectual and emasculated husband, while also bearing responsibility for influencing Ichiro's refusal to swear allegiance to the United States – a decision that leads to his two-year imprisonment. Mrs. Yamada further represents the lingering spectre of imperial Japan, refusing to acknowledge its defeat in World War II. However, as this denial collapses under the weight of reality, she descends into psychosis and ultimately ends her life in the family grocery store. Mrs. Yamada thus embodies a Japanese presence fundamentally unable to assimilate into the sociopolitical assemblage of 1950s America. She is framed as "a deviation from both sexual and gender norms," aligning her with the figure of the disloyal communist or the political subversive (D. Kim 66–67).

In an era when traditional gender roles were weaponized as "ammunition in the ideological Cold War" to uphold societal and familial structures (Hartmann 86), Mrs. Yamada's characterization as an anomaly is striking. Narratively, she is depicted as expendable – a subject reduced to an Agambenian bare life, whose elimination carries no moral or social consequences. Her ontological materiality deteriorates into an abject state of madness, rendering her unrecognizable and devoid of normative agency. She becomes a lingering remnant of uncomfortable memories haunting the United States, a stigmatized and shameful emblem of rupture, disability, and abnormality within the national narrative, particularly in its treatment of the no-no boys.

Mrs. Yamada's abject existence denotes the unresolved contradictions and internal disparities within the US assemblage of the 1950s. These unresolved tensions disrupt the cohesive narrative of a unified American identity, embodying what Deleuze refers to as "difference-in-itself." As the "shadow of reality" (Deleuze, *Difference and Repetition* 73), this difference fractures the ideological representations, symbolic identities, and spatial environments of post-war America. "Your mama is sick, Ichiro, and she has made you sick, and I am sick because I cannot do anything for her" (Okada 35), laments Mr. Yamada, acknowledging the family's position as a point of irreconcilable difference that cannot be integrated into the actor-network of Cold War family ideology.

Upon returning home, Ichiro perceives his mother as a degenerate symbol of his hometown, where "everything looked older and dirtier and shabbier" (7). This ethnic enclave, with the Yamada family at its centre, exists as a persistent difference-in-itself – a "Japan in America" that challenges the nation's ability to fully reconcile its history of exclusion and assimilation. This shadow of reality continuously re-emerges as an obscure site that the United States struggles to affirm, underscoring the unacknowledged heterogeneity and unresolved ruptures within its imagined identity as a unified nation. As Deleuze notes, these fractures signal the potential for an "affirmed world of difference" (74), even as they resist easy resolution.

For Ichiro, Mrs. Yamada represents a regressive past, while Emi symbolizes a forward-looking perspective and the possibility of reintegration into post-war American society. Emi plays a pivotal role in the narrative by offering Ichiro emotional and material support, including employment, as he navigates the challenges of life after incarceration. Her provision of sexual and emotional solace serves as an analogy for the post-war United States' ideological aspiration to integrate no-no boys into its social fabric. In contrast, Mrs. Yamada compels Ichiro to remain entrenched in his no-no boy identity, hindering his psychological autonomy and social development. Emi's empathetic gestures, such as offering Ichiro a job when he hesitates to sever ties with his Japanese family, stand in stark opposition to Mrs. Yamada's influence.

Okada's narrative juxtaposes the two women's physicality to underscore their ideological and symbolic roles (89). Mrs. Yamada is described as a "small, flat-chested, shapeless woman ... [with] the awkward, skinny body of a thirteen-year-old" (Okada 11), whereas Emi is portrayed as "a few inches taller than Kenji ... [and] slender with heavy breasts, had rich, black hair which fell on her shoulders and covered her neck." Emi's "long legs" are likened to being "strong and shapely like a white woman's" (77), highlighting a stark contrast. This juxtaposition reveals the eugenic epistemology embedded within Okada's ableist narrative, which aligns with the broader cultural and racial aesthetics of mid-century America (Zhang 89).

In the early twentieth century, US popular culture perpetuated "aesthetic propaganda" that valorized white, slender, and physically flexible bodies, reinforcing "eugenic constructions of fitness and defectiveness" within prevailing beauty standards (Pernick 91–92). As Yijing Zhang puts it, women of marginalized "gender, class, race, and ethnicity" were often categorized as unattractive or flawed, their perceived imperfections associated with disability (89). Simultaneously, American society confined women to narrowly defined gender and sexual roles, predominantly as wives and mothers. These archetypes – rooted in domesticity, child-rearing, and patriotic service – formed the basis of what in the 1960s Betty Friedan famously called the "feminine mystique" (7). Women were even cast as ideological buffers against perceived communist threats during the Cold War (Meyerowitz 241).

Okada's narrative projects this feminine mystique onto Emi's voluptuous body and compliant femininity, presenting her as an embodiment of idealized womanhood. Emi's alignment with traditional notions of female gender, body, and sexuality contrasts sharply with Mrs. Yamada, whose nonconforming physical and ideological traits mark her as an aberration within the post-war American landscape. This dynamic underscores the broader societal pressures to conform to normative roles and appearances, revealing the ableist and racialized undercurrents that shape the characters' identities and relationships.

The physical, sexual, and gender disparities between Mrs. Yamada and Emi invite scrutiny, particularly in the context of their portrayals as sacrificial figures of Japanese American women. Mrs. Yamada's pathological, disabled, and abject femininity disrupts conventional gender norms, contradicting the family ideology of the 1950s (Li 90–91). Lacking normative femininity, she emasculates her husband's patriarchal masculinity, reducing him to "a goddamned, fat, grinning, spineless nobody." Consequently, Ichiro perceives his mother as a relentless force, a "rock that is always hammering, pounding ... in her unobtrusive, determined, fanatical way until there's nothing left to call one's self" (Okada 13). Feeling crushed by his mother's overpowering disabled motherhood, Ichiro blames her for the court decision that led to his imprisonment, believing that it pushed him into "an emptiness that is ... more frightening than the caverns of hell." He curses her for what he perceives as cruelty and hatred, lamenting that he will never experience the meaning of life again (13). Daniel Kim argues that Ichiro falls victim to Mrs. Yamada's "momism," where the overpowering mother exerts unnatural control within the family (66). Ichiro goes further, stating that she has "lost all the characteristics of femininity" (Li 91), dismissing her as "neither woman nor mother" (Okada 21).

In contrast, Emi's Westernized embodiment evolves in alignment with the gender, sexuality, and femininity ideals of the 1950s. When Ichiro feels empty, Emi places her bare breasts on his face, prompting him to sob like an abandoned child and momentarily fill the void of motherhood (84). Despite her "yellow skin" as an Asian, Emi represents the material turn that reflects the era's family ideology and expectations of womanhood, particularly in reference to "the virtue of white femininity" (Zhang 90), through her Westernized body.

However, Emi's Westernized body is not the only aspect of her character that undergoes this material transformation in Okada's narrative. Her family relationships provide her with the opportunity to distance herself from her Japanese identity. Her Japanese parents, repatriated to Japan after the Pearl Harbor attack, express their discontent in a letter: "Sick. Sick of Japan and Japanese and rotten food and sicker still of having to stay there" (Okada 78). Additionally, her husband, Ralph, chooses to remain in Japan, refusing to return to America or reunite with Emi. Emi's position within her family is exceptional, as they fully identify as neither American nor Japanese. They exist in "the realm of irreducible ambiguity between outside and inside, between chaos and normality," a "state of exception" as described by Agamben (19). Within this state of exception, Okada's narrative portrays Emi as the only member of her family recognized as a chosen American, enjoying the privilege of survival within the 1950s US assemblage. Her inclusion in American political life contrasts with the fate of the rest of her family, who are consigned to the status of bare life and denied this privilege.

Emi's family saga illustrates how Japanese ontology is relegated to what Agamben describes as the state of exception, where individuals are deemed expendable and can be "killed with impunity" (72). This categorization reflects a perception of their materiality as unhealthy and unfit – qualities that the narrative seeks to erase from the Cold War image of post-war America. Like Mrs. Yamada, Emi's parents and her husband, Ralph, disappear from the 1950s American landscape, lacking the capacity for a material turn to integrate as proper Americans. Similarly, Okada's narrative excludes the Yamada family and other no-no boy Japanese families from the Cold War portrayal of the 1950s United States, which idealized families as "strong, stable, and self-reliable" (May 10). These un-American families are portrayed as deviant, abnormal, and disabled – incapable of embodying the security apparatus necessary for instilling American ideals of race, gender, and sexuality. Ichiro's resentment toward his mother is emblematic of this exclusion, as it leads him to reject and despise the "half" of himself that is Japanese (Okada 16). Through its ableist lens, the narrative leverages the immutable foreignness of Japanese heritage, devoid of potential for transformation, to rationalize the eugenic underpinnings of white supremacy.

In comparison, Emi represents an embodiment of the 1950s feminine mystique and successfully forges a symbiotic relationship with her white American neighbours. Her agency facilitates a material turn, transforming the disabled ontology of Japanese heritage into a normate American identity and contributing to Ichiro's eugenic assimilation into post-war America. She provides him with employment on her farm and helps him discover "a purpose in life" (87), symbolically aiding his departure from the regressive ties to his Japanese heritage. Emi underscores the necessity of choosing a single identity, telling Ichiro that it is impossible to be both American and Japanese simultaneously (84). She insists that America is "a big country with a big heart" and urges him to "be equally big, forgive [the country's mistakes], and be grateful to it." Emi's "pride and patriotism" for America reflect her belief that Japanese Americans can become "worthy of" belonging to the country (88). Through this guidance, Emi seeks to alleviate the "destructive mental consequences" (D. Kim 65) of Ichiro's past decisions, steering him towards acceptance and reintegration into the American ideal.

## The Yellow Body Ornamented with "a Bunch of Japs"

Anne A. Cheng introduces the concept of ornamentalism to examine how the femininity, gender, and sexuality associated with Asian women's bodies contribute to colonial knowledge within Western colonial discourse. She conceptualizes it as an additional decorative and intricate signifier imposed on the corporeality of Asian women at a superficial, physical level. These ornamental signifiers, Cheng argues, adorn the body with supplementary value, meaning, and imagery, facilitating its objectification, animalization, and fetishization. Through the fetishistic gaze of white men, the "yellow decorativeness" of colonized women's bodies is materialized in ways distinct from the fetishization of white women. This yellow body, embodying the "entanglement of organic corporeality and aesthetic abstraction," becomes further intertwined with epistemologies of non-humanity, such as animality and thingness. Cheng asserts that this ornamental skin "becomes – is – flesh for Asian American female personhood," highlighting how the white male gaze exploits the gendered, racialized, and sexualized inhuman materialities of yellow skin. This process transforms Asian women into aesthetic objects for consumption, resulting in a "(con)fusion between thingness and personness" (Cheng 14).

Although Cheng's primary focus is on Asian women, the dynamics she describes also extend to broader Orientalist constructions shaping perceptions of Asian masculinity. These align with Edward Said's Orientalism, which outlines how the West has historically represented the East as exotic, mysterious, and inferior. In this framework, Asian men have frequently been portrayed as effeminate, weak, and lacking normative masculinity. In the context of *No-No Boy*, Kenji's wounded leg becomes a potent symbol of the existential vulnerability and stigmatization of Japanese bodies in post-war America. His injury – a festering leg wound sustained in Europe during his service as a yes-yes boy fighting the Nazis – serves as a metaphor for the impending demise of Japanese ontology, deemed expendable and obsolete in the American cultural landscape.

Kenji copes with his injury through repeated amputations of the decaying portions of his leg at the Veterans Affairs hospital, enduring the physical pain in exchange for economic compensation and symbolic recognition as a normative citizen. His status as a war hero allows him to achieve a semblance of the American Dream, but his injured leg simultaneously embodies the material, corporeal, and symbolic stigma inscribed on his Asian body. The wound serves as both a marker of his sacrifice and a reminder of his exclusion from the idealized image of a normate American. Kenji's leg, as a site of symbolic castration, indicates the intersection of race, masculinity, and bodily vulnerability, challenging post-war America's assimilationist ideals and the purported universality of its citizenship.

Okada's narrative juxtaposes this physical and symbolic struggle against the backdrop of the 1950s idealized American family, defined by democratic and harmonious familial relationships. Kenji recounts to Ichiro a sociologist's speech he overheard in the internment camp, which questioned the inmates' ability to enjoy familial companionship: "How many of you are able to sit down with your own sons and daughters and enjoy the companionship of conversation?" (Okada 113). This observation reflects the era's family ideology, which sought to reframe the ornamentalized, racialized bodies of no-no boys into ethnically assimilated material acceptable to white Americans.

Kenji's family gathering before his final surgery further reinforces this idealized portrayal of middle-class American family life. His relatives, most of whom are professionals, exchange stories about everyday topics such as fishing, new cars, baseball games, the military, and insurance. This depiction of an affluent yet tranquil family environment serves as a quintessential representation of the 1950s American Dream. It highlights the cultural capital associated with middle-class life, emphasizing their successful assimilation and fulfilment of societal expectations – an accomplishment starkly absent in Ichiro's family.

Although both families share Japanese heritage, the disparity between them is accentuated through contrasting depictions of their patriarchs. Mr. Yamada is portrayed as an ineffectual figure, overwhelmed by crises such as his wife's insanity and suicide, Taro's assault on Ichiro and subsequent departure, and his own descent into alcoholism. In contrast, Kenji's father embodies the American ideal of masculinity. Described as "a big man, almost six feet tall and strong," he expresses empathy for his son's sacrifices and the resulting pain, demonstrating the qualities of a loving and communicative father (Okada 106). This stark contrast not only reflects the divergent trajectories of the two families but also stresses the narrative's alignment with assimilationist ideals tied to race, gender, and class in post-war America.

Hence, the narrative positions Kenji as having achieved the privilege and status necessary to embody the normate American ideal. He seems poised to represent the quintessential American, except for the inescapable foreignness of his Japanese body – an ornamental "yellow" corporeality that gradually deteriorates, undermining his otherwise American existence. This ornamental essence of his racialized body remains an unassimilable materiality, marked as unhealthy and unfit for the post-war US imaginary. Furthermore, the absence of a mother in Kenji's family, despite its alignment with other markers of middle-class respectability, precludes it from fully embodying the normative ideal of a 1950s American family. Kenji's commendable military service cannot override the symbolic weight of his deteriorating body. His decaying leg becomes an ontological residue of his marginalized identity, representing what he disparagingly terms "a bunch of Japs" (Okada 146) – a part of himself that post-war America seeks to either suppress or eliminate.

The term "Japs," much like Kenji's festering leg, signifies a difference-in-itself within the US assemblage, a locus of fear, pain, and despair etched onto the ornamental canvas of his yellow skin. This ideological interpellation relegates him to a state of exception, marking him and his Japanese peers with a stigmatic and traumatic negation that denies them the full realization of their American identity. Given this, Okada's ableist narrative functions as an ideological state apparatus, dramatized through the symbol of Kenji's decaying leg – a site of censorship and punishment for his racial and bodily affiliation with both the "Japs" and no-no boys. This inassimilable materiality, ultimately excised from Kenji, serves as a vanishing mediator that facilitates the uneasy reconciliation of his dual identity: an American G.I. and a racialized "Jap." The post-war United States emphasized the rehabilitation of disabled veterans, prioritizing the restoration of normative masculinity to signify national recovery and strength (Wu 5). However, in reality, many disabled veterans remained "outsiders, physically and psychologically cut off from the domestic abundance of American life" (Kinder 272).

Moreover, Kenji's disability, while adorned as a badge of honour from his service as a G.I., is also a marker of his racialized otherness. His yellow skin – metaphorically tied to his medical and racial disability – becomes an ornamental layer concealing the deeper societal rejection of his dual identity. Okada's narrative uses Kenji's impaired leg as a focal point, exposing how his physical and racialized disability symbolizes the Jap-materiality of negation and exclusion. Through this symbol, the narrative critiques the structural contradictions of post-war American ideals, where the promise of inclusion is persistently undermined by the realities of racial and bodily exclusion.

In Ichiro's eyes, the "medal, car, pension, [and] education" (Okada 55) that Kenji earned through his military service exemplify the possibility for a disabled individual with a Japanese body to ascend to the status of a first-degree American citizen. To Ichiro, Kenji embodies the ideal American, fully entitled to "the right to laugh, love, hope ... and to hold his head high" (58). In stark contrast, Ichiro perceives his own Japanese body as an "empty shell" (58), devoid of the fundamental attributes necessary for assimilation into normate American society. Caught between two identities, Ichiro exists as someone who is "neither Japanese nor

American" (68), a disenfranchised and disabled figure burdened by pathological emptiness, quiet sadness, and an insatiable hunger for purpose and belonging (53).

Kenji, in this context, becomes more than a friend; he is a benefactor who "feels for" (67) Ichiro, offering him tangible and symbolic gifts – a "new Oldsmobile," an introduction to Emi, and, most significantly, the hope of rediscovering a "purpose in life." These gestures provide Ichiro with tools to begin filling his "empty shell," a shell "stripped of dignity, respect, purpose, [and] honor" (12). In this way, Kenji functions as a vanishing mediator, a transitional figure who facilitates the potential for Ichiro's material turn – a transformative process through which Ichiro might reclaim agency and find a pathway toward integration into the American ideal, despite the lingering obstacles posed by his racial and cultural identity.

### Okada's Ableist Desire for a Transversal Turn from Japanese to American

In *No-No Boy*, Japanese Americans collectively bear the ornamental matter of their yellow bodies, symbolizing their perceived perpetual un-Americanness. Yet they remain caught in a continuous process of becoming American – a state of perpetual self-alienation that lies at the heart of Okada's ableist narrative. This narrative endeavours, albeit unsuccessfully, to eradicate the ingrained markers of otherness from the historical, ideological, and cultural memory of the 1950s. Kenji partially embodies this material turn as a disabled and doomed figure, slowly succumbing to his decaying leg – a physical manifestation of his racialized difference – through repeated amputations until his eventual death. While persistently dismissed as "just another Jap" (Okada 74), Kenji's transformation into a model minority teeters on the edge of assimilation, with his death at the Veterans Hospital symbolizing the culmination of his material turn. This turn is achieved only through the removal of the lethal Oriental leg, a symbolic rejection of his racialized body within the framework of Okada's ableist narrative.

Before his passing, Kenji leaves Ichiro with the bitter realization that any Nisei striving to become an "able-bodied" American will ultimately confront the same fate: "a little time to get cut down to their own size. Then they'll be ... a bunch of Japs" (141). This struggle to navigate the dual identity of being Japanese while proving otherwise underscores Kenji's tragic effort to attain a "point of wholeness and belonging" (138) as an American – a goal that ultimately costs him his life. Despite being described as a "Japanese who [is] more American than most Americans," Kenji's ultimate sacrifice for his country – a radical act of self-negation – reveals the futility of his aspirations for full acceptance. His material turn, while seemingly a step towards integration, is incomplete, marked by exclusion and mortality.

In Okada's narrative, Kenji and Ichiro are both reduced to the label of "a bunch of Japs," locked in the perpetual process of becoming disabled Americans, with their birthright to citizenship denied from the outset. Ichiro's lament – "Where is that place they talk of and paint nice pictures of and describe in all the home magazines ... where the families all have two children ... and a shiny new car in the garage ... like living in the land of the happily-ever-after?" – captures this exclusion poignantly (142). Neither Kenji nor Emi, nor Ichiro himself, achieves the status of a normate American, despite Kenji's middle-class affluence and Emi's embodiment of the 1950s feminine mystique. Instead, they remain trapped in what Ichiro calls a "rotten place, rotten and filthy and cheap and smelly" (142), existing on the margins of the American Dream. Thus, the narrative frames the Japanese body as analogous to the colonial subject, aligning with Deepika Bahri's description of the "native body split apart under imperial eyes" and "re-envisioned as a multiply disabled, dysplastic body, lacking in the collective and individual graces of civilization" (15). In this sense, the ornamental yellow corporeality of Japanese Americans is portrayed as inherently destined to perish unless it undergoes a transformative material turn – an act fraught with loss, erasure, and unfulfilled belonging.

Compared to Ichiro, Gary exemplifies a no-no boy who has undergone a more advanced transformative turn. Working at a Christian rehabilitation centre, he strives to evolve into a more transversal self, transitioning from his Japanese identity toward an American one. Reflecting on his personal journey, Gary openly admits, "I came back to life" after having "rotted in prison," noting that "old friends are now strangers" (Okada 198). His optimism persists as he emphasizes, "there are still plenty of good [white] people around" (200), citing Mr. Carrick as one such figure. Ichiro admires Carrick, a liberal-democratic white man whom Emi describes as the "kind of American that Americans always profess themselves to be" (151). However, Carrick embodies a guilt-ridden yet colourblind liberalism, paternalistically stating to Ichiro, "Eng for Eng, Jap for Jap, Pole for Pole, and like for like meant classes and distinctions and hatred and prejudice and wars and misery" (140–41).

Okada's narrative reflects the eugenic ableism pervasive in 1950s America, portraying Ichiro and Kenji as "Jap boys," permanently marginalized. In stark contrast to Gary's transformative trajectory is Freddie, another no-no boy who resists the era's norms of containment and integration. Freddie's defiance is encapsulated in his declaration, "Me,

I don't give a damn" (45). Lacking the prospect of eugenic improvement, Freddie rebels by pursuing a reckless affair with a married neighbour and ultimately meets a tragic end in a fatal car chase, a casualty of despair. Freddie symbolizes the rebellious no-no boy, whose self-destructive life, according to Okada's narrative, stems from his futile effort to vent the hatred of being labelled a "Jap" (Xu 59). Without the potential for an affective transversal turn, Freddie's fate embodies the narrative's ableist underpinnings.

The relationship between Kenji and Ichiro provides a dialectical lens to explore the existential crisis of Japanese Americans in the 1950s, shaped by white supremacy's ableist ideology. The two characters embody ambivalent yet interconnected facets of Japanese American identity: Kenji, the model minority who clings to a precarious life, and Ichiro, the suspended actor caught between two irreconcilable worlds. Despite their differences, both share the ornamental materiality of the Japanese body, described as "one already dead but still alive and contemplating fifty or sixty years more of dead aliveness, and the other, living and dying slowly" (68).

Through this synthesis of the yes-yes and no-no boy archetypes, Okada's narrative examines the future of Japanese America. Ichiro's seemingly hopeless pursuit of a normate identity hinges on a faint "glimmer of hope," while Kenji's trajectory, emblematic of the model minority, teeters towards a premature end. Their divergent yet parallel lives underscore the existential plight of Japanese Americans in the post-war era. Kenji's material demise signifies not just the loss of his life but also the erasure of his Japaneseness, while Ichiro remains in a perpetual state of exception, suspended between Japanese and American identities. Both characters ultimately inhabit positions of disabled subjectivity, excluded from the ableist ideal of a "wholly America" (66). This vision of wholeness and belonging is predicated on the continuous (re)production of marginalized figures, like the no-no boys, to uphold the American ideal.

## Conclusion: Home as "No Place in Particular"

Okada's *No-No Boy* portrays the historical journey of Japanese Americans navigating the post-war US "empire of feeling" (D. Kim 77) – a complex matrix of white supremacy, containment, liberal democracy, and Cold War Orientalism. As the United States transitioned into a liberal democratic empire with a transpacific orientation, Okada's narrative critiques the intertwined systems of racism, ableism, sexism, classism, socialism, and capitalism that shaped the 1950s. The novel also functions as a confessional exploration of lived experience, interrogating whether the antinomic (un)presence of people of Japanese descent could ever be fully absorbed into mainstream American society. In this context, Okada offers a historical narrative of transformation, tracing how the "disabled matter" of Japan in America was gradually reconstituted into the normative fabric of American identity during a period of geopolitical realignment in which Japan shifted from wartime adversary to Cold War ally.

The novel concludes with Ichiro leaving his hometown, pursuing "that faint and elusive insinuation of promise" (221) in his quest to fill his "empty shell" and achieve a state of being "wholly American." His uncertain trajectory mirrors the real-life experiences of many no-no boys. For example, Toru Saito, who spent four years in the Topaz internment camp in Utah, returned there regularly. In a 1988 interview during one such visit, he remarked, "Going back there helps me define who I am, recharges my batteries, and gives me a sense of my own identity" (Saito). Similarly, Sharon Yamato, reflecting on her release from the Manzanar internment camp in 1949, said, "In the four short days it took to dismantle these barracks, I touched the silent pain of my parents' lives. At Heart Mountain, I took a hammer and tore down a wall" (Yamato).

Many Japanese Americans continue to make pilgrimages to these camps, honouring both the collective and individual histories embedded in these spaces. Such visits preserve memory while asserting identity. Lawson F. Inada's poem "Manzanar" encapsulates this duality, describing the camps as a distinctive part of Japanese American identity: "This is a part of our enduring geography. This is a part of who we are. No one can take that away" (Inada). For Inada, the camps exist as sites of both trauma and existential significance, places Japanese Americans feel compelled to revisit. Deprived of their homes during internment, many found no other place to return to after their release. Like Kenji in the novel, Okada himself was a war veteran. When asked by his superior in Guam, where he had begun his military service, where he was from, Okada reportedly replied, "No place in particular" (*No-No Boy* xxvi). This response captures the pervasive dislocation experienced by Japanese Americans in the post-war period. Although Okada died before the rediscovery and republication of *No-No Boy* in 1971, it seems likely that he, too, spent the remainder of his life searching for a sense of belonging and a home that had been irretrievably lost.

## WORKS CITED

Abe, David K., and Allison Imamura. "The Destruction of Shinto Shrines in Hawaii and the West Coast during World War II: The Lingering Effects of

Pearl Harbor and Japanese-American internment." *Asian Anthropology*, vol. 18, no. 4, 2019, pp. 266–81. https://doi.org/10.1080/1683478X.2019.1592816.

Agamben, Giorgio. *Homo Sacer: Sovereign Power and Bare Life*. Stanford UP, 1998.

Amoko, Apollo O. "'Resilient Imaginations': *No-No Boy*, *Obasan* and the Limits of Minority Discourse." *Mosaic: A Journal for the Interdisciplinary Study of Literature*, vol. 33, no. 3, 2000, pp. 35–55.

Bahri, Deepika. *Postcolonial Biology: Psyche and Flesh after Empire*. U of Minnesota P, 2017.

Benjamin, Ruha. *Race after Technology: Abolitionist Tools for the New Jim Code*. Polity, 2019.

Chen, Tina. *Double Agency: Acts of Impersonation in Asian American Literature and Culture*. Stanford UP, 2005.

Cheng, Anne A. *Ornamentalism*. Oxford UP, 2019.

Dalrymple, Louis. "School Begins." *Puck. The Forbidden Book: The Philippine-American War in Political Cartoons*, edited by Abe Ignacio et al., T'Boli, 2004.

Deleuze, Gilles. *Difference and Repetition*. Translated by Paul Patton, Columbia UP, 1994.

Deleuze, Gilles and Claire Parnet. *Dialogues II*. Translated by Hugh Tomlinson and Barbara Habberjam, rev. ed., Columbia UP, 2007.

Deleuze, Gilles and Félix Guattari. *Anti-Oedipus: Capitalism and Schizophrenia*. Translated by Robert Hurley et al., U of Minnesota P, 1983.

–. *A Thousand Plateaus*. U of Minnesota P, 1987.

Fanon, Frantz. *The Wretched of the Earth*. Grove, 2005.

Friedan, Betty. *The Feminine Mystique*. Dell, 1974.

Hartmann, Susan M. "Women's Employment and the Domestic Ideal in the Early Cold War Years." *Not June Cleaver: Women and Gender in Postwar America, 1945–1960*, edited by Joanne Meyerowitz, Temple UP, 1994, pp. 84–176.

Inada, Lawson Fusao. "Manzanar." *The Manzanar Pilgrimage: A Time for Sharing*, edited by Manzanar Committee. Manzanar Committee, 1981, pp. 38–40, https://www.asianamericanbooks.com/books/3230.htm.

Jonnes, Denis. *Cold War American Literature and the Rise of Youth Culture: Children of Empire*. Routledge, 2015.

Kim, Chang-Hee. "The Cold War Biopolitics of Disability in John Okada's *No-No Boy*: Racialized and Gendered Ableism of American Society in the 1950s." *Modern Fiction in English*, vol. 29, no. 2, 2022, pp. 77–111. https://doi.org/10.22909/smf.2022.29.2.004

Kim, Daniel Y. "Once More, with Feeling: Cold War Masculinity and the Sentiment of Patriotism in John Okada's No-No Boy." *Criticism*, vol. 47, no. 1, 2005, pp. 65–83.

Kinder, John M. *Paying with Their Bodies: American War and the Problem of the Disabled Veteran*. U of Chicago P, 2015.

Kipling, Rudyard. "The White Man's Burden." *The Literature Network*. 1899. 18 Sept. 2012

Klein, Christina. *Cold War Orientalism: Asia in the Middlebrow Imagination, 1945–1961*. U of California P, 2003.

Kogawa, Joy. *Obasan*. Anchor, 1994.

Li, Wenxin. "An Untenable Dichotomy: The Idea of Home in John Okada's *No-No Boy*." *Asiatic*, vol. 9, no. 1, 2015, pp. 81–93.

Ling, Jinqui. "Race, Power, and Cultural Politics in John Okada's *No-No Boy*." *American Literature*, vol. 67, no. 2, 1995, pp. 359–81. https://doi.org/10.2307/2927793.

Lowe, Lisa. *The Intimacies of Four Continents*. Duke UP, 2015.

Malmgren, Carl D. "Texts, Primers, and Voices in Toni Morrison's *The Bluest Eye*." *Critique*, vol. 41, no. 3, 2000, pp. 251–73. https://doi.org/10.1080/00111610009601590

May, Elaine Tyler. *Homeward Bound: American Families in the Cold War Era*. Basic Books, 1988.

–. "'Family Values': The Uses and Abuses of American Family History." *Revue Française D'études Américaines*, vol. 3, no. 97, 2003, pp. 7–22.

Meyerowitz, Joanne. "Beyond the Feminine Mystique: A Reassessment of Postwar Mass Culture, 1946-1958." *Not June Cleaver: Women and Gender in Postwar America, 1945–1960*, edited by Joanne Meyerowitz, Temple UP, 1994, pp. 229–62.

Morrison, Tony. *The Bluest Eye*. Vintage, 2007.

Nielsen, Kim E. *A Disability History of the United States*. Beacon Press, 2013.

Ng, Wendy L. *Japanese American Internment during World War II: A History and Reference Guide*. Greenwood Publishing Group, 2002.

Nguyen, Viet Thanh. *Race and Resistance: Literature and Politics in Asian America*. Oxford UP, 2002.

Okada, John. *No-No Boy*. U of Washington P, 1976.

Ozeki, Ruth. Forward. *No-No Boy*. U of Washington P, 1976, pp. vii–xviii.

Pereira, Malin Walther. "Periodizing Toni Morrison's Work from *The Bluest Eye* to Jazz: The Importance of Tar Baby." *MELUS*, vol. 22, no. 3, 1997, pp. 71–82. https://doi.org/10.2307/467655

Pernick, Martin S. "Defining The Defective: Eugenics, Esthetics, And Mass Culture In Early Twentieth-Century America." *The Body and Physical Difference: Discourses of Disability*, edited by David T. Mitchell and Sharon L. Snyder. University of Michigan Press, 2000, pp. 89–110.

Rand, Naomi R. *Roth, Morrison and Silko Studies in Survival*. 1995. City U of New York, PhD dissertation.

Said, Edward W. *Orientalism*. Pantheon, 1978.

Saito, Toru. From a display in the Japanese American National Museum, Los Angeles, California. 23 Jun. 2019.

Shinoda, Michael Kenji. "Kenji-Fort Minor." *YouTube*, uploaded by Fort Minor, 31 Aug. 2010, https://www.youtube.com/watch?v=pUBKcOZjX6g.

Song, Min Hyoung. *The Children of 1965: On Writing, and Not Writing, as an Asian American*. Duke UP, 2013.

Thiong'o, Ngugi wa. *Decolonising the Mind: The Politics of Language in African Literature*. James Currey, 1986.

Winfield, Ann Gibson. *Eugenics and Education in America: Institutionalized Racism and the Implications of History, Ideology, and Memory*. Peter Lang, 2007.

Wu, Cynthia. "'Give Me the Stump Which Gives You the Right to Hold Your Head High' – A Homoerotics of Disability in Asian Americanist Critique." *Amerasia Journal*, vol. 39, no. 1, 2013, pp. 3–16. https://doi.org/10.17953/amer.39.1.j65431864q72gp28.

Xu, Wenying. "Sticky Rice Balls or Lemon Pie: Enjoyment and Ethnic Identities in *No-No Boy* and *Obasan*." *Literature Interpretation Theory*, vol. 13, no. 1, 2002, pp. 51–68. https://doi.org/10.1080/10436920210419.

Yamato, Sharon. From a display in the Japanese American National Museum, Los Angeles, California. 23 Jun. 2019.

Zhang, Yijing. *The Cold War Construction of Dis/abled Asian Bodies in Transpacific Asian American Literature*. 2021. Yonsei U, PhD dissertation.

Zimmerman, Eugene. "There Is an Old 'Yank' Who Lives in a Shoe." *Judge*. New York. 13 August 1989. *The Forbidden Book: The Philippine-American War in Political Cartoons*, edited by Abe Ignacio, et al. T'Boli. 2004.

# PART II

# Queering Embodied Health Narratives

# 4 Vaccination, Pandemics, and Fear in the Now

SANDER L. GILMAN

In the "good old days," we in the medical humanities (today rethought as the health sciences humanities) used to blithely speak of *metanarratives* (pace Jean-François Lyotard and, in a different way, Hayden White) – overarching stories that provided clear answers to complex problems. With the work of Sara Ahmed and Laura Otis, we now understand that such metanarratives have the force of containing and focusing our emotional responses to the past in the light of our assumed relationship to that past. Our question has become *how* do we instrumentalize the history of the NOW? Hans Ulrich Gumbrecht, well in advance of our age of plague, noted that "different from the ever shrinking and therefore 'imperceptibly short' present of the historicist chronotope, the new present (that continues to be our present in the early twenty-first century) is one in which all paradigms and phenomena from the past are juxtaposed as being available and ready-to-hand. For this present, instead of leaving the past behind, is inundated with pastness" (Gumbrecht 271). Constituting that pastness means focusing our emotional response in the present through our need to posit a usable past. This can, on a material level, seem to echo what Stephen Hinchliffe et al. have described as the *terrains of infectability*: "the planetary aspect of this condition of so-called infectability (ie, the extent to which an organism is vulnerable to becoming infected). This focus includes linking the emergence of SARS-CoV-2 and similar novel viruses to habitat destruction, illegal trade in wild animals, climate instabilities, and changing intensities of the relationships between humans and other animals" (e232).

But all these contemporary concerns in the *now* mask an underlying anxiety, triggered by the need to posit the source of fear beyond the self. This is the underlying focus of the moral panic that defines Western notions of what Paula Treichler in the age of HIV/AIDs called a "semantic plague." For example, my colleague Zhou Xun and I, in our recent study of this problem, dealt with the so-called "bush-meat" debate evoked in Hinchliffe et al.'s litany of linked material "realities" in the world of pandemic in our study of xenophobia and pandemics, as it is a claim that linked HIV/AIDs to SARS to COVID-19. Whether these are "real" in the material sense seems secondary to the fact that the exoticism of eating practices different from one's own is an immediate locus for the fears triggered by these pandemics. We wouldn't eat such things – *they* do – but now *we* are at risk! (Zhou and Gilman 43ff)

The touchstone for all Western (and postcolonial) texts representing plague, the generic forerunner of our anxiety about pandemic, remains Thucydides' fifth-century BCE *History of the Peloponnesian War*. It is the Meta – or at least the Ur-narrative on mass death, from whatever physiological cause. As we remember from our college readings of the Great Books, after the second invasion of the Peloponnesians the Athenians underwent a change of feeling, now that their land had been ravaged a second time by Sparta while the plague and the war combined wreaked havoc at home as earthquakes rattled the windows of their houses. They blamed Pericles for having persuaded them to go to war and held him culpable for all misfortunes that had befallen them. Thucydides, a general during the war, speaks about the plague as well as the social disorder from, he states, his own experience: "I shall describe its actual course, explaining the symptoms, from the study of which a person should be best able, having knowledge of it beforehand, to recognize it if it should ever break out again. For I had the disease myself and saw others sick of it" (Thucydides 342–43). But who was really at fault? Maybe the Africans or the enemies who poisoned the wells? (The evocation of this during the Black Plague, a millennium or so too later, targeted Jews and undertakers!): "The disease began, it is said, in Ethiopia beyond Egypt, and then descended into Egypt and Libya and spread over the greater part of the King's territory. Then it suddenly fell upon the city of Athens, and attacked first the inhabitants of the Piraeus, so that the people there even said that the Peloponnesians had put poison in their cisterns; for there were as yet no public fountains there" (Thucydides 343).

You will notice how careful Thucydides is with the hearsay about its origins, noting that both the Ethiopians and the Peloponnesians were accused – "it is said" – and yet why was it so necessary to place the origin of the plague so far from the responsibility of the citizens of Athens?

What the multiyear plague caused was fear, unfathomable, exquisite fear. And this fear could not be ameliorated by the usual appeals to the healers. It seemed to be necessary to question why medicine, and

Athens had a complex guild of healers who linked religious belief and medical theory as well as praxis, were unable to achieve any means of amelioration:

> And no one remedy was found, I may say, which was sure to bring relief to those applying it – for what helped one man hurt another – and no constitution, as it proved, was of itself sufficient against it, whether as regards physical strength or weakness, but it carried off all without distinction, even those tended with all medical care. And the most dreadful thing about the whole malady was not only the despondency of the victims, when they once became aware that they were sick, for their minds straightway yielded to despair and they gave themselves up for lost instead of resisting, but also the fact that they became infected by nursing one another and died like sheep. And this caused the heaviest mortality; for if, on the one hand, they were restrained by fear from visiting one another, the sick perished uncared for, so that many houses were left empty through lack of anyone to do the nursing; or if, on the other hand, they visited the sick, they perished especially those who made any pretensions to goodness. (Thucydides 349, 351)

The political response heard from Pericles shouting to the crowd to assuage their fear was more or less "Make Athens Great Again":

> I am well aware that your displeasure with me has been aggravated by the plague; but there is no justice in that, unless you mean to give me also the credit whenever any unexpected good fortune falls to your lot. ... But the right course is to bear with resignation the afflictions sent by heaven and with fortitude the hardships that come from the enemy; for such has been the practice of this city in the past, and let it find no impediment in yourselves. ... And realize that Athens has a mighty name among all mankind because she has never yielded to misfortunes, but more freely than any other city has lavished lives and labours upon war, and that she possesses to-day a power which is the greatest that ever existed down to our time. (Thucydides 370)

Then Pericles too perished in the plague.

Medical practice in Athens was overwhelmed by the plague (Longrigg; Mitchell-Boyask). The healers could not heal; the temples offered little solace. Ritual burials were abandoned, corpses were denied funerary rites and, at a certain point, were simply dumped helter-skelter in mass graves. A few years later, during a truce in the Peloponnesian War, some Athenians imported the cult of Asclepius, son of Apollo and the

Greek god of healing. Asclepius, whose name means "to cut open," was cut from his dead mother's womb by his father, Apollo. It was, of course, Apollo in the guise of Apollo Acesius ("the healer"), whose temple on the Agora came to be filled with the dead and dying during the plague; and who thus was believed to be on the side of the Spartans. Among Asclepius's daughters were Hygeia (health and sanitation), the mother of the public's health, and Panacea (cure all), the godmother of all quacks. The cult of Asclepius was established towards the end of the sixth century BCE at Epidaurus, located in the Peloponnesus across the Saronic Gulf from Athens. Early during the plague, Athens had attacked Epidaurus, presumably with the goal of acquiring the cult by force. By the end of the plague, around 420 BCE, the Athenians constructed a sanctuary of the healing god Asclepius next to the Theatre of Dionysus on the south slope of the Acropolis. And a new medical guild enters Athenian society, the priest of Asclepius. What is striking about the new cult is that it relied as much on demanding the longer-term presence of the person seeking healing, as they performed the rite of incubation, which meant sleeping in the temple, hoping for a miraculous cure, awaiting a dream that encoded a cure in some form. It was not merely giving an offering and leaving; this transformed the temple into a place of psychic as well as physical healing (Hamilton 8-44). As one recent commentator has observed: "Following the devastation of the plague, the Athenians began reestablishing norms and supportive institutions. The rise of the cult of Asclepius can be a social movement that featured redemptive religious healing and a reformative political strategy. In addition, the rise of the cult paralleled the emergence of the Asclepiad physicians and Hippocratic writings that date between 427 and 400 BCE. This aspect of the movement influenced the development of western scientific medicine" (Perlstadt 1051).

And given the centrality of dreams in the therapy, alternatives to even our understanding of scientific medicine. Given that the so-called Hippocratic Oath is introduced during the lead-up to scientific medicine, in the age of secularized medical instruction beginning in the nineteenth century, this seems to be doubly true. But the great ancient healers that followed in the Greco-Roman world, Pliny, Galen, and Aetius, do more than acknowledge the primacy of Hippocratic medicine, in the tradition of which they stood if centuries later; they created the legend that Hippocrates had "fought the epidemic by building a great fire, which corrected the unhealthy atmosphere that caused the outbreak" (Pinault 53). And that was "a flat contradiction of Thucydides' statement that physicians were helpless against the disease and were often themselves the first victims. That doctor was the fabled Hippocrates"

(Pinault 52). Plague pandemics demand some means of framing fear, even in the past, whether by physicians, public health experts, politicians, or priests. After Thucydides, the physicians insisted that there had been some successes and who better to choose than the deified Hippocrates of Kos, the old healer healing in the past. Thucydides' account of the plague not only highlighted the physicians' failure but framed it in the collapse of societal norms, norms that provide physicians and patients with tools to deal with their fears.

Thucydides observed the resultant social collapse of Athenian society, including any faith in the healers, as "the plague first introduced into the city a greater lawlessness. For where men hitherto practiced concealment, that they were not acting purely after their pleasure, they now showed a more careless daring. ... No fear of gods or law of men restrained; for, on the one hand, seeing that all men were perishing alike, they judged that piety and impiety came to the same thing" (352).

Under normal times, Thucydides opines, we are just fine; this was an awful time, and our emotions got the better of our Athenian rationality (Orwin). Fear defined the response to the plague, but equally importantly, it defined our narrative of the plague, as Thucydides' attempt to locate its origin "over there" in the world of the Ethiopians was a way of identifying the source of our fear. Once identified as beyond our scope, it became something that appeared from outside and therefore could well disappear outside again.

Let us move now to seventeenth-century Great Britain, in a world as racked by catastrophe as that of Thucydides or indeed our own. Not only plague but civil war and massive fires brought the fear of dissolution into each person's daily life. Of all the commentators on catastrophe in the time, Thomas Hobbes was most clearly the continuation of *The Greeks* in his role as the first English translator of Thucydides' *History of the Peloponnesian War* (1629), with its account of the Athenian plague, a plague blamed by Thucydides on the Ethiopians, as well as the simultaneous wars that undermined Athenian life. Hobbes later writes in his *Leviathan* (1651), as we all can quote, that life in its natural setting was a war "of every man against every man ... and which is worst of all, continuall feare, and danger of violent death; And the life of man, solitary, poore, nasty, brutish, and short" (Hobbes, *Leviathan* 63), all well in advance of 1665, with the Great Plague followed in 1666 by the Great Fire of London, both startling only in their scope, not in their unfamiliarity.

Hobbes's narrative reflected fear, fear of the collapse of civil society. Only the government can save us from our own permanent entropy – unlike Thucydides, who thought that human irrational responses were a permanent reaction to catastrophe but were recuperable once order was restored and time had passed. *We do not learn from the plague or anything else!* shouted Hobbes; these catastrophes only reveal what we really are under the veneer of civilization. And Abraham Bosse's frontispiece of Hobbes's *Leviathan* showed us why. He depicts, in its central panel, two plague doctors, with full PPE (at least for the seventeenth century, including beaked masks) walking the streets of an abandoned cityscape (Falk). The individual voluntarily submits to the fear of the law and to the terror of the "public sword" to avoid such worlds. It is "freedom from" in the Hobbesian sense of "liberty," unfettered action of human beings living in what he imagined to be a state of nature that needed to be controlled. "Liberty" (we might say licence) is understood by him as the absence of interference with any of one's actions. But true freedom demands in the end an accountability to the collective, freedom limited to substantially protect those in your world from harm, if possible. Thomas Hobbes sees that by each subsuming themselves to the power of the political community, they are rescued from the terrors of such "liberty," where "there is perpetual war of every man against his neighbour; no inheritance to transmit to the son, nor to expect from the father; no propriety of goods or lands; no security" (140). And we can add random exposure to death and social displacement from plague, something with which Hobbes would have been well acquainted, as friends and patrons had died of the plague. Such a view was very personal for Hobbes in the time of plague, as Sterling P. Lamprecht observed:

> While many Englishmen were prone to blame the fire on those whom they considered the "treacherous Catholics," the plague was obviously an act of God. The House of Commons shared this widespread attitude and, desirous of ridding the country of the causes of the divine displeasure, named several persons whose wickedness might be the occasion of the display of God's wrath against the English people. The House included Hobbes in the list and specifically mentioned his Leviathan. Moreover, some bishops of the Church of England, at about the same time, suggested that it might be well to burn Hobbes as a heretic. (31)

The underlying assumption is that we remain irrational beings and that catastrophes in the NOW only reveal our underlying irrationality, especially when we are targeted as the very cause of these catastrophes. While, as H. L. Mencken wrote about the Spanish Flu, we can suppress memory: "The epidemic is seldom mentioned," he wrote in the 1920s, "and most Americans have apparently forgotten it." "This is not surprising," he added. "The human mind always tries to expunge the intolerable from memory, just as it tries to conceal it while current" (qtd. in Collier 304). Yet forgetting and remembering demand models for both. We turn to the Greeks for a tale about the plague, as well as evoke their image of the River Lethe to apostrophize forgetting. Instrumentalizing history, using the metanarratives we can retrieve from the past, shapes our emotional responses in the now.

By the Enlightenment, Hobbes clearly dominated, at least in the world of law. Sir William Blackstone's eighteenth-century commentary on British jurisprudence, annotating the 1603 law on plague under James I, summarized how the administrative state inculcated that fear of the "public sword":

> any person infected with the plague, or dwelling in any infected house, he commanded by the mayor or constable, or other head officer of his town or vill, to keep his house, and shall venture to disobey it; he may be enforced, by the watchmen appointed on such melancholy occasions, to obey such necessary command: and, if any hurt ensue by such enforcement, the watchmen are thereby indemnified. And farther, if such person of commanded to confine himself goes abroad, and converses in company, if he has no plague fore upon him, he shall be punished as a vagabond by whipping, and be bound to his good behaviour: but, if he has any infectious fore upon him uncured, he then shall be guilty of felony.

The notion that the state had the primary obligation, despite all calls for individual "liberty," in the Hobbesian sense to at least attempt to control the spread of disease was well established even before more modern views of the dangers of infectious diseases to the public's health. One can acknowledge that state interventions will never be foolproof against an infectious pathogen, but the absence of any such enforceable state or collective actions almost guarantees its spread.

As we now know, John Locke had his copy of Thomas Hobbes's *Leviathan* on his virtual night table and ascribed individual "freedom" as his answer to the notion of the obligation of the state to correct for the self-destructive actions of individuals (Waldmann). Locke is in dialogue with Hobbes but brackets in a complex way the obligation of the state in times of plague. Locke's experience of the Great Plague was coloured by his understanding of miasma theory that epidemic disease resulted from natural circumstances, such as drought bringing forth effluvia hidden within the earth (following Robert Boyle), as well as Sydenham's Hippocratic notion that each epidemic was unique in its manifestations. Both systems, to quote Thomas Sydenham, "depend upon certain hidden and inexplicable changes within the bowels of the earth" (Dewhurst 321). Thus, human activity, such as that which Locke commented on in Paris, Orleans, and Languedoc, could neither limit nor moderate the cause of plague and marked the limitations of all medical interventions. This meant that Locke avoided proscribing the activities of the individual in such circumstances. What Blackstone, and indeed most legal systems, recognize is that the state has an interest in preserving the overall health of its citizens. Even when the means it undertakes may not be efficacious. Blackstone's mid-eighteenth-century views had a formative influence on the writing of the American Constitution in 1787 and subsequent legal theory and practice. Among the absolute rights he advocated were "the right of personal security [that] consists in a person's legal and uninterrupted enjoyment of his life, his limbs, his body, his health, and his reputation" (Blackstone).

Remember that Blackstone was the *Common Law for Dummies* in the American colonies and that lawyers, like Thomas Jefferson reading law at the College of William and Mary from 1760 to 1762, knew this text backwards and forwards. It is striking that when Jefferson penned the Declaration of Independence in 1776, he translated Blackstone's rights into Lockean terms: "that all men are created equal, that they are endowed by their Creator with certain unalienable Rights, that among these are Life, Liberty and the pursuit of Happiness. – That to secure these rights, Governments are instituted among Men, deriving their just powers from the consent of the governed." *Health* vanishes as that could not be the result of the consent of the governed, only the action of the state (Miles et al.).

But starting in the early twentieth century, the age of a more detailed understanding of the science of infectious diseases, American constitutional law holds that the states may pass and enforce laws that are intended to control the spread and eradication of epidemics. These findings build on quarantine laws that are present from the earliest findings in American law. In constituting the symbolic register for the national community, health (here defined as combating disease) is an absolute defining aspect of community identity. Disease/health is one of the factors that defines the "boundaries" of the nation state, certainly by the Enlightenment dissolution of the notion of a divine state and ruler created by God. In Benedict Anderson's widely cited *Imagined Communities: Reflections on the Origin and Spread of Nationalism* (1983), he argues that communities as such arise when the national state needs a symbolic register; the flag, the leader, language, race, or indeed, health and illness come to be the focus of the newly constituted "natural" symbolic community. Anderson writes, "in everything 'natural' there is always something unchosen. In this way, nation-ness is assimilated to skin-colour, gender, parentage, and birth-era – all those things one cannot help. And in these 'natural ties' one senses what one might call 'the beauty of gemeinschaft.' To put it another way, precisely because such ties are not chosen, they have about them a halo of disinterestedness" (47). Here the symbolic overlay of the idea of population health (or illness) becomes yet one more "disinterested factor," which is, on the contrary, a highly invested manner of defining the community.

Here is the conflict: if one of the state's obligations to the collective is managing plague, what happens to the "pursuit of liberty"? Isaiah Berlin's famous definition of negative "freedom from" state control in his 1958 lecture on "Two Concepts of Liberty" is coupled with a view of "freedom to" – the notion that state actors, pace Hobbes, Blackstone, and Anderson, have an obligation to provide limits on individual action. "What is the area within which the subject – a person or group of persons – is or should be left to do or be what he is able to do or be, without interference by other persons?" whereas we use the positive concept in attempting to answer the question "What, or who, is the source of control or interference that can determine someone to do, or be, this rather than that?" (Berlin). For as Isaiah Berlin notes, the defender of positive freedom will take an additional step that consists of conceiving of the self as wider than the individual and as represented by an organic social whole – "a tribe, a race, a church, a state, the great society of the living and the dead and the yet unborn" (Berlin 132). "Once I take this view," Berlin says, "I am in a position to ignore the actual wishes of men or societies, to bully, oppress, torture in the name, and on behalf, of their 'real' selves, in the secure knowledge that whatever is the true goal of man ... must be identical with his freedom" (Berlin 133). Berlin has the Nazis and the Soviets in mind, not *public health* authorities. *But* what if the bullying intended to mitigate pandemics leads to actions that infect and kill? On the part of those who follow public health guidelines (magic thinking kills) or deny them (as does resistance to them), the arch-liberal legal scholar Cass R. Sunstein and his arch-conservative colleague at Harvard Law Adrian Vermeule, during the age of COVID-19, argued that there is a necessity of a Hobbesian perspective for a proactive state in their defence of the administrative state, labelling this as "the morality of administrative law": "those who support the administrative state deny that it is a threat to liberty, properly understood. Consider some of the actual activities of that state. Would people be freer without child labor laws? ... Without protection against pandemics? Some defenders of the administrative state argue that it is not only constitutionally permissible, but also in some sense mandatory, if the goal is to carry into execution the promises of the constitutional scheme" (Sunstein and Vermeule 5).

This debate evokes all the earlier discussion of state control and plague. The touchstone is notions of risk and choice, but as we well know, all concepts of choice have an affective dimension. In the NOW, vaccination has been a touchstone for debates about "freedom" or "liberty" since Edward Jenner introduced vaccination to replace variolation in 1789. With variolation, there was a heightened risk of infection and death, which was assumed to be eliminated, rather than ameliorated, with the new use of cowpox. As we know George III's son, Octavius, died of smallpox following his variolation and his ghost haunted his father's madness. That would, it was assumed, vanish with the new procedure, as we are now confronted with a rational choice between health and illness. Vaccines thus come to be a test case for liberty, as in the premiere case in American jurisprudence, *Jacobson v Massachusetts*. The Swedish-American pastor Henning Jacobson, living in Cambridge, argued that subjecting him to a fine or imprisonment for neglecting or refusing vaccination for smallpox, mandated by the Commonwealth of Massachusetts, was an invasion of his liberty, that the law was "unreasonable, arbitrary and oppressive," and that one should not be subjected to the law if he or she objects to vaccination, no matter the reason. The courts held with Hobbes, not Locke: "Even liberty itself, the greatest of all rights, is not an unrestricted license to act according to one's own will. It is only freedom from restraint under conditions essential to the equal enjoyment of the same right by others. It is then liberty regulated by law.... Real liberty for all could not exist under the operation of a principle which recognizes the right of each individual person to use his own [liberty], whether in respect of his person or his property, regardless of the injury that may be done to others" (*Jacobson v Massachusetts* 196–97).

The case was smallpox, a deadly disease which claimed as many as 15 million victims in 1967 but, because of its successful eradication in 1980, no longer frames the debate in the twenty-first century.

Now we can move our discussion of microbes and plague to a more recent *now*. By the beginning of the twenty-first century, state mandated mass vaccinations were ubiquitous. Smallpox had been eradicated globally, and in developed states epidemic diseases such as polio and early childhood infectious diseases were rare if not non-existent. The anti-vax movement, which had been marginal and limited mainly to religious and political fringe groups after Jacobson, had become mainstream and middle class, "soccer moms" not Norwegian ministers. By 2005 there was the strong suggestion that Jacobson, the case and the person, was now deceased. Wendy K. Mariner and her colleagues argued that, in our enlightened Lockean age: "Public health programs that are based on force are a relic of the 19th century; 21st-century public health depends on good science, good communication, and trust in public health officials to tell the truth. In each of these spheres, constitutional rights are the ally rather than the enemy of public health. Preserving the public's health in the 21st century requires preserving respect for personal liberty" (581, 588), Such an argument is only possible in a world that has forgotten or repressed smallpox, polio, and other diseases that were part and parcel of the fabric of the state's self-identity. But it also revealed the great divide still existing between Hobbes and Locke. They do not consider the affective dimension of public health. They assume that the "man on the Clapham Omnibus" aka the American "man on the street," the Australian "man on the Bondi tram," the Canadian "person on the Yonge Street subway" is a Reasonable Man.

Here the generic *man* does represent a fantasy of a rational and logical *person* in a logical and rational patriarchal culture. Women, as I have shown in many of my earlier works on the notion of hysteria, are the test case for unreasonableness (Gilman et al.). In the 1930s, in A. P. Herbert's account of the hypothetical case of *Fardell v Potts*, the court held that as common law does not mention a "reasonable woman":

> The view that there exists a class of beings, illogical, impulsive, careless, irresponsible, extravagant, prejudiced, and vain, free for the most part from those worthy and repellent excellences which distinguish the Reasonable Man, and devoted to the irrational arts of pleasure and attraction, is one which should be as welcome and as well accepted in our Courts as it is in our drawing-rooms – and even in Parliament. The odd stipulation is often heard there that some new Committee or Council shall consist of so many persons "one of which must be a woman": the assumption being that upon scientific principles of selection no woman would be added to a body having serious deliberative functions. That assumption, which is at once accepted and resented by those who maintain the complete equality of the sexes, is not founded, as they suppose, in some prejudice of Man but in the considered judgments of Nature. I find that at Common Law a reasonable woman does not exist. (Herbert 34)

Neither, of course, does a "reasonable man."

A reasonable man is a "fictional" or "notional" person (*Nova Mink v Trans-Canada Airlines*). Justice James Laidlaw of the Ontario Court of Appeal aptly described him in the 1950s as:

> a mythical creature of the law whose conduct is the standard by which the Courts measure the conduct of all other persons and find it to be proper or improper in particular circumstances as they exist from time to time. He is not an extraordinary or unusual creature; he is not superhuman; he is not required to display the highest skill of which anyone is capable; he is not a genius who can perform uncommon feats, nor is he possessed of unusual powers of foresight. He is a person of normal intelligence who makes prudence a guide to his conduct. He does nothing that a prudent man would not do and does not omit to do anything a prudent man would do. He acts in accord with general and approved practice. His conduct is guided by considerations which ordinarily regulate the conduct of human affairs. His conduct is the standard "adopted in the community by persons of ordinary intelligence and prudence." (*Arland and Arland v Taylor*)

The court cited the original definition of 1856 by Justice Edward Hall Alderson (the Victor Frankenstein of law?) who created the reasonable man and therefore furnished common law world with a "natural" definition of negligence:

> Negligence is the omission to do something which a reasonable man, guided upon those considerations which ordinarily regulate the conduct of human affairs, would do, or doing something which a prudent and reasonable man would not do. The defendants might have been liable for negligence, if, unintentionally, they omitted to do that which a reasonable person would have done, or did that which a person taking reasonable precautions would not have done. (*Blythe v Birmingham Waterworks Co*)

In fact, A. P. Herbert, in his caricature of the reasonable man, goes further in attributing a personality – and perhaps neuroses – to the man who navigates the world with a self-conscious awareness of the implications of his every actions, "who invariably looks where he is going, and is careful to examine the immediate foreground before he executes a leap or bound; who neither star-gazes nor is lost in meditation when approaching trap-doors or the margin of a dock; who never mounts a moving omnibus, and does not alight from any car while the train is in motion" (31). He writes of the reasonable man that he never

> swears, gambles, loses his temper, ... does nothing except in moderation, and even while he flogs his child is meditating on the golden mean. Devoid, in short, of any human weakness, with not one single saving vice, sans prejudice, procrastination, ill-nature, avarice, and absence of mind, as careful for his own safety as he is for that of others, this excellent but odious

creature stands like a monument in our Courts of Justice, vainly appealing to his fellow citizens to order their lives after his own example. (Herbert 32)

Indeed, A. P. Herbert did not miss the role of disease either. In a later comic case illustrating "An Act of God" defining this as "something no reasonable man could have expected" (317), the relative awareness of the potential cause of damages is seen as defining. The argument hinges not on the scope of the disaster, such as an earthquake, but its ramifications: "I can conceive that a widespread epidemic of plague or infectious fever might be held to be an Act of God, though caused by a single minute and invisible bacillus" (Herbert 317). That the aged, retired judge hearing the matter had stepped in for five colleagues down with the influenza certainly was intended to colour the reference. (Herbert 453) Thucydides and Hobbes, looking at human nature in the age of plague, understood that this fantasy of a reasonable man was a veneer, easily pierced by external events.

Wendy K. Mariner et al.'s paper demanding a revision of laws concerning vaccination came because of Merck in November 2004 unveiling a vaccine called Gardasil for certain strains of human papillomavirus (HPV), a precursor of cervical cancer (Lindén). The pharmaceutical giant marketed it as a cervical cancer vaccine for "girls." The CDC approved the new vaccine, unanimously for vaccination of girls and women 11 to 26 years. Now, who is affected by HPV? The population initially targeted by Gardasil was young women. To this point, the intent was to "protect" this specific population. The two most carcinogenic types of HPV, HPV16 and HPV18, that the vaccine protected against are associated with about 70 percent of cervical cancers. In the United States during 2007, there were about 13 000 new cases of cervical cancer and 4021 deaths from the disease. This was a radical decrease over 40 years because of Pap smears and early detection.

But the right wing said immediately in light of the availability of the vaccine: HPV is a STI! Abstinence is the only way to prevent HPV, they argued. In a hearing concerning HPV vaccines in Congress in 2004, Dave Weldon, a physician and then a Republican representative from Florida, stated:

While the CDC is to be commended for promoting abstinence as a sure means to avoid HPV infection, it has taken a long time for this common sense and science-based conclusion to be reached.

Other agencies have been quick to spend some $6 billion on research to advance methods of identifying and treating cervical cancer but little on

> true primary prevention and risk avoidance. I believe that this inattention to abstinence as a positive public health approach is only a symptom of a larger, more troubling phenomenon, a phenomenon that places science behind politics and social agendas....
>
> We have known for years that STDs, including HIV/AIDS and HPV, are closely associated with promiscuous sexual behavior. But most of our public health approaches have sought to employ intervention modalities to reduce the rate of infection instead of true prevention strategies. Instead of seeing reductions in HIV/AIDS, Chlamydia, and HPV, we have seen significant increases year after year. (*Hearing before the Subcommittee*)

But even more than that, maybe the vaccine is not safe for this vulnerable population, as an anti-abortion group claimed:

> The National Vaccine Information Center (NVIC) is calling on the CDC's Advisory Committee on Immunization Practices (ACIP) to just say "no" on June 29 to recommending "universal use" of Merck's Gardasil vaccine in all pre-adolescent girls. NVIC maintains that Merck's clinical trials did not prove the human papillomavirus (HPV) vaccine designed to prevent cervical cancer and genital warts is safe to give to young girls. "There is too little long term safety and efficacy data, especially in young girls, and too little labeling information on contraindications for the CDC to recommend Gardasil for universal use, which is a signal for states to mandate it ... Nobody at Merck, the CDC or FDA know if the injection of Gardasil into all pre-teen girls – especially simultaneously with hepatitis B vaccine – will make some of them more likely to develop arthritis or other inflammatory autoimmune and brain disorders as teenagers and adults. With cervical cancer causing about one percent of all cancer deaths in American women due to routine pap screening, it was inappropriate for the FDA to fast track Gardasil. It is way too early to direct all young girls to get three doses of a vaccine that has not been proven safe or effective in their age group. ("Merck's Gardasil Vaccine")

Is the risk from a treatment for a STI worth undertaking? Or should we demand social controls such as universal condemnation of (premarital) sexual activity. The voices on the then fringe Right continued, as they had in opposition to MMR vaccination of infants and claimed that Gardisal caused retardation: "Rep. Michelle Bachmann, of Minnesota, raised that concern by suggesting that Mr. Perry had put young girls at risk by forcing "an injection of what could potentially be a very dangerous drug." She recounted that after the debate in Tampa, Florida, a tearful mother approached and said her daughter had suffered "mental retardation" after being vaccinated against HPV. "It can have very dangerous side effects" (Gabriel and Grady). Was this risk treating people who caused their own misery by their lack of sexual control? Liberty or license?

Yet in February 2007, the ultraconservative Governor of Texas, Rick Perry, mandated the vaccine: "The HPV vaccine does not promote sex, it protects women's health. In the past, young women who have abstained from sex until marriage have contracted HPV from their husbands and faced the difficult task of defeating cervical cancer. This vaccine prevents that from happening" (Blumenthal). Premarital abstinence is no panacea as reprobate men violate the marriage bed because of their lack of self-control. The Libertarians, such as the then "Representative Ron Paul of Texas [an MD with an OB/GYN specialty before he entered politics] aggressively challenged Mr. Perry on several fronts, including for pushing through an executive order requiring young girls to have an inoculation against a sexually transmitted disease, HPV, before reversing course. 'This is not good medicine, I do not believe,' he said. 'It's not good social policy. And therefore, I think this is very bad to do this'" (Zeleny and Nagourney). The state legislature of Texas agreed with Paul and disagreed with the governor, overturning the state's requirement for vaccination in April 2007. The Texas experience had a chilling effect across the country. In early 2007, HPV vaccine mandates were pending in most state assemblies in the country. To date, no state has passed an HPV mandate.

Gardasil was marketed like the vaccine for hepatitis B. In the 1980s, there were about 200 000 to 300 000 new cases of hepatitis B in the United States each year, with most infections spread through unprotected sex or intravenous drug use. No Pap smear ameliorated the results of the infection, and the most troubling aspect of the virus was that it can later cause liver cancer. So, when it was developed in 1981, the hepatitis B vaccine was touted by the manufacturer as the "first effective anti-cancer vaccine ever developed." As a sexually transmitted infection, hepatitis B is qualitatively different from the archetypal disease (smallpox) for which vaccination is required. It is highly contagious, but it is not airborne. Hepatitis B epidemics can and do occur because many carriers are unaware that they have the disease and do not or will not take proper precautions. In 1981 a vaccine against *cancer* was unique and was one of the goals of the "War Against Cancer" declared by Richard Nixon in 1971, a moment still in the aura of the new polio vaccines. The difference between the social status of the cancers of hepatitis B and those of HPV seemed to be not the means of transmission or the infectious potential of the virus but the organ that was impacted:

livers seemed much less easy to moralize about than vaginas (Hesketh; Mukherjee).

The general sense was that the fear associated with the very word *cancer* was a more successful selling point for both the hepatitis B and the HPV vaccine. We know well from the public health literature that the very word *cancer* creates a fear that colours its origin or even its treatability (Dresser). CANCER BAD! is the Western mantra. In the general American population, the fear of cancer seems to have trumped the debate about chastity or vaccination among young women. As of 2022, 100 million had received at least one dose of Gardasil. About 54.2 percent of teens in the United States were fully vaccinated against HPV. Roughly 56.8 percent of girls were up to date on HPV vaccination, up from 53.7 percent in 2018. It seems that the idea of a "cancer" vaccine has taken hold to protect what is often described as a "vulnerable" population, despite the protests of those who oppose vaccination or premarital sex. This extraordinary success has meant that Gardasil, then the only cervical cancer vaccine on the market, has made US$1.5 billion in sales since 2006.

But wait – moralizing aside, HPV really is an STI! It is transmitted through vaginal or anal sexual contact and fulfils all the categories applied to STIs in public health. In this sense, it is little different from the newest and virulent outbreaks of treatment-resistant syphilis. It clearly impacts the women who have the virus as they may well develop cervical cancer. But, like syphilis, it can also damage their offspring. Recurrent respiratory papillomatosis (RRP), which is the result of being infected with HPV in the birth canal, causes blockage of the airway, damaged vocal cords, lung damage. It can lead to multiple surgeries and it can lead to death. Newborn children, like the women of Rick Perry's Texas, are vulnerable people. In the population that has HPV infections, about 1 in 400 deliveries results in the infection being spread to the newborn baby who can develop RRP; there are about 2000 new cases of RRP a year in the United States. The HPV vaccine also prevents damage to children born to women who may have no idea that they are infected with the virus or that they are placing their child at risk of lifelong, chronic illness.

Now who is impacted by this infection based on this rhetoric: certainly "vulnerable populations" such as infants and women are, especially "innocent" women in Texas. "Vulnerability" is, however, a very slippery label. Some recent theories of law (as in the work of Martha A. Fineman) see this as an overarching, neutral, and universal term, rather than labels such as *disabled* or *aged* or *marginalized*: "Vulnerability is posited as the characteristic that positions us in relation to each other as human beings and also suggests a relationship of responsibility between state and individual" (Fineman 255). Public health constantly re-writes what it thinks are "vulnerable populations," trying to empirically define these as those most "at-risk" in any given situation (Shi and Stevens). Vulnerability is a term that is always coded by what a society fears most about its own weakness, its assumed points of fragility, its own fantasies of the antithesis of vulnerability, which brings us, of course, back to the problem of a "reasonable man." Thus, the at-risk populations seem to be those exposed to HPV that cause cervical cancer in "girls" infected by (*disgusting*) diseased men, especially in Texas, and *innocent* children suffering from RRP caused by these same men.

But men are vulnerable people too, as I boldly stated in a paper in *The Lancet* in 2009:

> Men too are a vulnerable population at risk from the deadly results of HPV infections. Recently, the steep increase in oral cancers among men has been traced to an increase in HPV infections stemming from the equal practice of oral sex by both sexes; from 1973 to 2004 oral cancers associated with HPV infections became about as common as those from tobacco and alcohol and today they are increasingly seen as their primary cause. Perhaps we should begin advocating Gardasil for young men who are also at risk from catastrophic illnesses resulting from HPV infection caused by women? (Gilman 1421)

By 2011 HPV was seen as the most important cause of the radical increase in throat and buccal cavity (oropharyngeal) cancers. Sexual practices, already long before Bill Clinton's claim that "he did not have sex with that woman," had shifted radically, and mutual oral-genital contact had become more commonplace. As a result, in the 1980s HPV was found in only 16 percent of the throat cultures of those with cancer – but in 72 percent of those collected after 2000. Anil K. Chaturvedi and her colleagues documented in 2011 that throat cancers caused by the virus increased to 2.6 per 100 000 people in 2004 from 0.8 cases per 100 000 people in 1988. If the trend continued, they argued, by 2020 the virus would be causing more throat cancer than cervical cancer (Chaturvedi et al., "Human Papillomavirus"). And to their credit their later work bore this out, even with the introduction of vaccine and herd immunity (Chaturvedi et al., "Prevalence of Oral HPV," "Oral Leukoplakia"). What happens in a highly charged political world, where fear is defined by human sexuality, is that the debates about vaccination come to be read as moral debates about sexual practice. Cancer, which is a potential result of such infections in *all* people, turns out in this context to be a more morally acceptable target for public health interventions than the vector of the transmission of the infection that may be its cause. Indeed, Gardasil television advertisements in 2023 still stressed a wide range of cancers as the reason for all to be vaccinated for HPV.

We began with fear and plague, with Thucydides and Hobbes, and end with the need to ask hard questions about boundaries and placing blame, either on the Ethiopians, on the Catholics, or indeed on men. This debate hung on the central fact that we always make decisions based not on "facts" and "rational" choice, but on the affect associated with this in any given context. Thus, a note in the *Harvard Law Review* in 2008, during the struggle to understand HPV vaccination as a public health/moral problem attempted to thread the needle:

> Vaccine law distinguishes between two kinds of necessity – what this Note calls "medical necessity" and "practical necessity." Those vaccines classified as "medically necessary" would be those that are the only known viable defenses against diseases taking hold in a community. "Practically necessary" vaccines are those to which there are alternatives, but which alternatives are, in practice, not used by a significant number of people.... for sexually transmitted diseases (STDs) like HPV, compulsory vaccination is not a medical necessity because individuals can protect themselves through some combination of sexual knowledge, disease screening, safe sex, and abstinence. But vaccination may still be necessary in practice if people do not take adequate precautions, and legally compelled immunization is the only practical way to combat the disease effectively. Of course, the line between medical and practical necessity will not always be clear. ("Rational People?")

The reasonable man strikes again: if only people acted in their own best interests. The line is certainly not clear; indeed, it really does not exist, if we translate this into the debates about COVID-19 and think about masking as facial condoms, with all of the moral force advocating for and against both. Think of vaccination as a medical necessity or a breach of individual freedom. Jefferson was so very wise to leave this debate out of his draft. Can we not simply, as Richard H. Thaler and Cass R. Sunstein do, "nudge" people by a "libertarian paternalism" into taking the "right" course by allowing a small number of opt-outs in the debate about HPV (Sunstein and Thaler)?

But they miss the point as we now see in the second age of Trump, where Harvard's Adrian Vermeule, in 2025 a member of the Trump administration, joyously heralds the dissolution of the administrative state, undertaken in part by the anti-vaxxer Robert F. Kennedy Jr., now heading the Department of Health and Human Service in a world of diminishing rate of vaccinations and new outbreaks of once rare contagious diseases. They, and those engaged in this debate even more violently with COVID-19, miss the point by assuming there are two players: the state and the individual, "control" or "liberty." But there is a third player who has equal agency: the virus. Bruno Latour illustrated this in his account of Louis Pasteur and anthrax:

> Pasteur adds to all the forces that composed French society at the time a new force for which he is the only credible spokesman – the microbe. You cannot build economic relations without this 'tertium quid' since the microbe, if unknown, can bitter your beer, spoil your wine, make the mother of your vinegar sterile, bring back cholera with your goods, or kill your factotum sent to India. You cannot build a hygienist social movement without it, since no matter what you do for the poor masses crowded in shanty towns, they will still die if you do not control this invisible agent. You cannot establish even innocent relations between a mother and her son, or a lover and his mistress, and overlook the agent that makes the baby die of diphtheria and has the client sent to the mad house because of syphilis. You do not need to muckrake or look for distorted ideologies to realize that a group of people, equipped with a laboratory – the only place where the invisible agent is made visible – will easily be situated everywhere in all these relations, wherever the microbe can be seen to intervene. If you reveal microbes as essential actors in all social relations, then you need to make room for them, and for the people who show them and can eliminate them. Indeed, the more you want to get rid of the microbes, the more room you should grant Pasteurians. This is not false consciousness, this is not looking for biased world views, this is just what the Pasteurians did and the way they were seen by all the other actors of the time. (Latour 157)

In the world of COVID-19, the virus is ubiquitous and omnipresent; yet simultaneously does not exist or exists only because of a conspiracy, a conspiracy of the pharmaceutical industry, of the laboratory at the Wuhan Institute of Virology, of Bill Gates, of the 5G networks. Like the state and the individual, the microbe has its own agency, for good or for ill. We can, of course, anthropomorphize this, as we regularly do with the "state," but the reality is that the debates about intervention only work when we see the virus as active and working towards its own goal, a goal that we might categorize as a "selfish gene," to plagiarize Richard Dawkins's account of the human being as merely a vessel for reproduction. Irrationality, human or microbial, is not part of the equation. We fear as part of who we are, but also who we are is shaped by where we are in time, space, and social structure. How we constitute the responses to our fears may exacerbate or diminish the fear and (perhaps) its causes, sometimes in productive and sometimes in destructive ways.

## WORKS CITED

Ahmed, Sara. *The Cultural Politics of Emotion*. Edinburgh UP, 2004.

Anderson, Benedict. *Imagined Communities: Reflections on the Origin and Spread of Nationalism*. Verso, 1983.

*Arland and Arland v Taylor*, 1955 CanLII 145, [1955] OR 131 at 142 (CA).

Berlin, Isaiah. "Two Concepts of Liberty" *Four Essays on Liberty*. Oxford UP, 1969, pp. 118–72. https://cactus.utahtech.edu/green/B_Readings/I_Berlin%20Two%20Concpets%20of%20Liberty.pdf.

Blackstone, William. *Commentaries on the Laws of England*. https://avalon.law.yale.edu/18th_century/blackstone_bk4ch13.asp. Accessed 2 Mar. 2022.

*Blyth v Birmingham Waterworks Co.* [1856], 11 Ex. 781 at 784.

Blumenthal, Ralph. "Texas Is First to Require Cancer Shots for Schoolgirls." *The New York Times*, 3 Feb. 2007, https://www.nytimes.com/2007/02/03/us/03texas.html.

Chaturvedi, Anil K., et al. "Human Papillomavirus and Rising Oropharyngeal Cancer Incidence in the United States." *The Journal of Clinical Oncology*, vol. 32, 2011, pp. 4294–301, https://doi.org/10.1200/JCO.2011.36.4596, Medline:21969503.

–. "Prevalence of Oral HPV Infection in Unvaccinated Men and Women in the United States, 2009–2016." *JAMA*, vol. 322, 2019, pp. 977–79, https://doi.org/10.1001/jama.2019.10508. Medline:31503300.

–. "Oral Leukoplakia and Risk of Progression to Oral Cancer: A Population-Based Cohort Study," *Journal of the National Cancer Institute*, vol. 112, 2020, pp. 1047–1054, https://doi.org/10.1093/jnci/djz238, Medline:31860085.

Collier, Richard. *The Plague of the Spanish Lady: The Influenza Pandemic of 1918-1919*. Macmillan, 1974.

Dewhurst, Kenneth. "A Review of John Locke's Research in Social and Preventive Medicine." *Bulletin of the History of Medicine*, vol. 36, 1962, pp. 317–40.

Dresser, Rebecca, editor. *Malignant: Medical Ethicists Confront Cancer*. Oxford UP, 2012.

Falk, Francesca. *Eine gestische Geschichte der Grenze: Wie der Liberalismus an der Grenze an seine Grenzen kommt*. Wilhelm Fink, 2011, pp. 63–90.

Fineman, Martha A. "The Vulnerable Subject and the Responsive State." *Emory Law Journal*, vol. 60, 2010, pp. 251–77, https://scholarlycommons.law.emory.edu/elj/vol60/iss2/1

Gabriel, Trip, and Denise Grady. "In Republican Race, a Heated Battle Over the HPV Vaccine." *The New York Times*, 14 Sept. 2011, https://www.nytimes

.com/2011/09/14/us/politics/republican-candidates-battle-over-hpv-vaccine.html.

Gilman, Sander L. "Human Papillomavirus, Abstinence, and the Other Risks." *The Lancet*, vol. 373, 25 Apr. 2009, pp. 1420–21, https://doi.org/10.1016/s0140-6736(09)60810-2, Medline:19400001.

Gilman, Sander L., et al. *Hysteria: A New History*. U California P, 1993.

Gumbrecht, Hans Ulrich. "Philology and the Complex Present." *Florilegium*, vol. 32, 2015, 273–81, https://doi.org/10.3138/flor.32.011.

Hamilton, Mary. *Incubation or The Cure of Disease in Pagan Temples and Christian Churches*. W. C. Henderson and Son, 1906.

*Hearing before the Subcommittee on Criminal justice, drug policy and human resources of the committee on government reform*. 108th Congress, 2nd Session. Serial no. 108-206, 11 Mar. 2004, https://www.congress.gov/event/108th-congress/house-event/LC14028/text

Herbert, A. P. *The Uncommon Law*. Eyre Methuen, 1952.

Hesketh, Robin. *Betrayed by Nature: The War on Cancer*. Palgrave Macmillan, 2012.

Hinchliffe, Stephen, et al. "Planetary Healthy Publics after COVID-19." *The Lancet: Planetary Health*, vol. 5, Apr. 2021, pp. e230–36, https://doi.org/10.1016/S2542-5196(21)00050-4, Medline:33838738.

Hobbes, Thomas. *Leviathan, or the Matter, Forme and Power of a Commonwealth Ecclesiastical and Civil*, edited by Michael Oakeshott, Oxford UP, 1960.

–. *History of the Peloponnesian War – Thucydides: The Complete Hobbes Translation*, edited by David Grene, U of Chicago P, 1989.

*Jacobson v Massachusetts*, 197 U.S. 11 (1905). https://supreme.justia.com/cases/federal/us/197/11/. Accessed 2 Mar. 2022.

Lamprecht, P. Sterling. "Hobbes and Hobbism." *American Political Science Review*, vol. 34, 1940, pp. 31–53, https://doi.org/10.2307/1948860.

Latour, Bruno. "Give Me a Laboratory and I Will Raise the World." *Science Observed: Perspectives on the Social Study of Science*, edited by Karin D. Knorr-Cetina and Michael Mulkay, Sage, 1983, pp. 141–69.

Lindén, Lisa. *Communicating Care: The Contradictions of HPV Vaccination Campaigns*. Arkiv Academic Press, 2016.

Longrigg, James. "The Great Plague of Athens." *History of Science*, vol. 18, 1980, pp. 209–25.

Mariner, Wendy K., et al. "Jacobson v. Massachusetts: It's Not Your Great-Great-Grandfather's Public Health Law." *American Journal of Public Health*, vol. 95, 2005, pp. 581–90, https://doi.org/10.2105/AJPH.2004.055160, Medline:15798113.

Miles, Albert S., et al. "Blackstone and His American Legacy." *Australia & New Zealand Journal of Law & Education*, vol. 5, 2000, pp. 46–59.

Mitchell-Boyask, Robin. *Plague and the Athenian Imagination: Drama, History and the Cult of Asclepius*. Cambridge, UP, 2008.

Mukherjee, Siddhartha. *The Emperor of All Maladies: A Biography of Cancer*. Simon & Schuster, 2010.

*Nova Mink v Trans-Canada Airlines*, [1951] 2 DLR 241, 26 MPR 389, 66 CRTC 316.

Orwin, Clifford. "Stasis and Plague: Thucydides on the Dissolution of Society." *Journal of Politics*, 50, 1988, pp. 831–47, https://doi.org/10.2307/2131381.

Otis, Laura. *Banned Emotions: How Metaphors Can Shape What People Feel*. Oxford UP, 2019.

Perlstadt, Harry. "The Plague of Athens and the Cult of Asclepius: A Case Study of Collective Behavior and a Social Movement." *Sociology and Anthropology*, vol. 4, 2016, pp. 1048–53, https://doi.org/10.13189/sa.2016.041203.

Pinault, Jody Rubin. "How Hippocrates Cured the Plague." *Journal of the History of Medicine and the Allied Sciences*, vol. 41, 1986, pp. 52–75, https://doi.org/10.1093/jhmas/41.1.52.

"Rational People? Toward a Twenty- First- Century *Jacobson v. Massachusetts*." *Harvard Law Review*, vol. 121, 2008, pp. 1820–41.

Sheppard, Jane. "Merck's Gardasil Vaccine Not Proven Safe for Little Girls." *Healthy Child*, 27 June 2006, https://healthychild.com/mercks-gardasil-vaccine-not-proven-safe-for-little-girls/.

Shi, Leiyu, and Gregory D. Stevens. *Vulnerable Populations in the United States*. 3rd ed., Jossey-Bass, 2021.

Sunstein, Cass R., and Adrian Vermeule. *Law and Leviathan: Redeeming the Administrative State*. Harvard UP, 2020,

Sunstein, Cass R., and Richard H. Thaler. "Libertarian Paternalism Is Not an Oxymoron." University of Chicago Law and Legal Theory Working Paper No. 43, 2003. https://chicagounbound.uchicago.edu/cgi/viewcontent.cgi?article=1184&context=public_law_and_legal_theory

Thucydides. *History of the Peloponnesian War*. Vol. I. Edited and translated by C. F. Smith. Harvard UP, 1919. Loeb Classical Library 108.

Treichler, Paula. "AIDS, Homophobia, and Biomedical Discourse: An Epidemic of Signification." *October*, vol. 43, 1987, pp. 31–70, https://doi.org/10.2307/3397564.

Waldman, Felix. "John Locke as a Reader of Thomas Hobbes's *Leviathan*: A New Manuscript." *Journal of Modern History*, vol. 93, no. 2, 2021, pp. 245–82. https://doi.org/10.1086/714068.

Zeleny, Jeff, and Adam Nagourney. "Perry and Romney Joust Over Direction of G.O.P." *The New York Times*, 8 Sept. 2011. https://archive.nytimes.com/query.nytimes.com/gst/fullpage-9F07E3DC163DF93BA3575AC0A9679D8B63.html.

Zhou, Xun, and Sander Gilman. *"I Know Who Caused COVID-19": Xenophobia and Pandemics*. Reaktion Press, 2021.

# 5 The Embodied Experience of Queer Moments: Crossing the Symptomatic Aesthetics of Joris-Karl Huysmans, Hervé Guibert, and David Wojnarowicz

BENJAMIN GAGNON CHAINEY

## Introduction

I propose to explore the embodied experiences of "queer moments," happening "when things fail to cohere" (Ahmed 170), in specific scenes of a syphilis and decadent writing from the end of the nineteenth century, in comparison to two AIDS and queer writings from the end of the twentieth century. To do so, I will complement Sara Ahmed's queer phenomenology with performativity theory, mainly Judith Butler's queer bodies that matter, Lee Edelman's queer death drive, and Judith Halberstam's queer art of failure. With that theoretical apparatus, I will explore how the comparison of different embodied experiences staged in the writings of both *fin de siècle*, can offer a new critical perspective on the symptomatic *aesthetics* of "queer moments," happening when sensations and spacetimes collide and disorient the affected and suffering bodies. Here, *aesthetics* is etymologically understood as "of or for perception by the senses, perceptive." Therefore, specific moments from *Against the Grain*, the cult novel of the decadent and symbolist movement, published by Joris-Karl Huysmans in 1884, will be compared to specific moments of Hervé Guibert's first two books about his suffering from AIDS – *To The Friend Who Did Not Save My Life* (1990) and *The Compassion Protocol* (1991) – as well as David Wojnarowicz's provocative writing about coming of age in America during the AIDS crisis, *Memories That Smell Like Gasoline* (1992). The chapter will focus on the aesthetic transformation of the characters' bodily symptoms into literary symbolism, in the different scenes. A key analytical concept that will guide my reading is that of *symptom*, a notion that is etymologically "altered from Late Latin *symptoma*, from Greek *symptoma* 'a happening, accident, disease,' from stem of *sympiptein* 'to befall, happen; coincide, fall together'" ("Symptom (n.)"). Accordingly, my analysis will follow four main questions: (1) How can the characters' embodied experience of queer moments be critically approached through the *aesthetics* of their different *symptoms*? (2) How do those different symptoms of sensory failure performatively disorient the bodies in space and time? (3) How do queer moments of symptomatic failure and disorientation, then, not only make the characters' human bodies become objects but also deploy new paths of signification through the style of their literary symbolism? (4) Finally, how does a critical approach anchored in queer aesthetics – of which, as Halberstam states it, "the darkness becomes a crucial part" (96) – allow a better understanding of the phenomenology and performativity of queer moments of disorientation, suffering and resurging trauma?

It is important to note, from the outset, that significant differences exist not only in terms of the genre of the works – *Against the Grain* being a pure phantasmagorical fiction, while Guibert's "AIDS writings" are commonly viewed as realistic autofiction, while Wojnarowicz's *Memories* can be situated more in the field of autobiography. The protagonists of the scenes that will be studied, consequently, are not of the same nature. The narrators Guibert and Wojnarowicz can be considered as the alter egos of their authors. However, *Against the Grain*'s anti-hero, Jean Floressas des Esseintes, cannot be considered as the (auto)biographical representation of an actual neurotic suffering from syphilis in the tertiary phase. The bringing together of those three characters – Des Esseintes, Guibert, and Wojnarowicz – and, more specifically, of the embodied experiences that they live *in the texts*, cannot give rise to a political critique that would be contextualized and coherent, given that their relationship to reality is not comparable. What they share, though, is their *textual* reality, rather than their historical and political context. I think it is legitimate to assert that ethical and political critiques of literary works currently dominate the disciplinary field and, even more markedly, the health humanities, which, in addition to their analyses of works, aim to improve the quality of care and health equity. Also, it's important to underline that renowned philosophers have brilliantly explored the ideological and political dimensions of the aesthetic approaches of art and literature. Indeed, since the rich theorization of aesthetics by Theodor Adorno, at the turn of the 1970s, several contributions have focused on the ideological character of aesthetic interpretation. Let us think in particular of the book by Terry Eagleton, aptly titled *The Ideology of the Aesthetic*, or the essay by Jacques Rancière, "The Politics of Aesthetics: The Distribution of the Sensible," translated in 2013, ten years after the publication of his version original, that rightly addresses the unequal distribution of the sensible, so as not to say the luxury of having the time and financial resources to reflect sensitively on the subjective effects caused by a work of art.

Although it is capital to address political inequity issues as a society, and as privileged academics, I believe it should not be the only focus of literary expertise, and it will *not* be the target of this chapter, which aspires – if this is still possible – to conduct its comparative analysis of scenes in the light of categories of aesthetics that are not directly related to political issues.

The goal is to focus on the performativity of the symptoms *felt* and experienced by the characters' *bodies in the texts*, to understand how their symptoms affect and disorient their sensitivity, and not how their experiences translate, tacitly or explicitly, into ethical and political issues of their respective time. Indeed, one could say that I pursue an aesthetic approach in *anachronistic counterpoint* to the approaches currently dominating the field, and this is precisely, perhaps, the political dimension of my approach: reconnecting with an aesthetic analysis giving primacy to the *quality of bodily sensations* – the *how* sensations are felt – even the most atrocious ones, rather than what they imply in their respective sociopolitical contexts.

What is more, it is important to emphasize that, apart from Wojnarowicz, known for his activism, notably alongside Nan Goldin, Huysmans and Guibert have both explicitly disengaged from any form of activism linked to the symptoms that they featured in their texts: those of syphilis for Huysmans and AIDS for Guibert. In the case of Huysmans, *Against the Grain* even went so far, in 1884, as to cause a radical break between its author and the naturalist movement, whose leader, Émile Zola, called on Huysmans to "set about studying morals" (Huysmans, *À Rebours* 65; my translation of "[m']atteler à une étude de mœurs" in "Préface écrite vingt ans après le roman") after his confusing and eccentric novel. As for Guibert, Didier Lestrade clearly criticized him for his lack of political commitment, in a chapter entitled "Against Guibert" (Lestrade 307) in his *History of Act Up*, published in 2000. In fact, even before he tested positive for HIV, and even if he very openly claims his homosexuality in his texts, at a time when it was still relatively taboo, Guibert bluntly states: "I am not a militant" (Guibert, *L'Image Fantôme* 89; my translation of "je ne milite pas").

In *The Politics of Aesthetics: The Distribution of the Sensible*, Rancière states: "The arts only ever lend to projects of domination or emancipation what they are able to lend to them, that is to say, quite simply, what they have in common with them: bodily positions and movements, functions of speech, the parceling out of the visible and the invisible" (19). It would be the work of a lengthy dissertation to enlighten what would be the common "emancipation project" of Huysmans, Guibert, and Wojnarowicz, considering the important spatio-temporal and sociological differences between them, as they cover together more than a century and two very different countries (France and the United States). Nevertheless, through various close readings of scenes, the chapter will contribute to the effort by precisely analyzing the multiple bodily positions and movements the protagonists are following in the texts. Given these few considerations, I want to insist on one point: aesthetic analyses focused on bodily symptoms do not necessarily *exclude* the political issues to which they could open, they are *complementary to them*. Is a reminiscence caused by a gustatory synesthesia or is a painful swallowing – as it will be discussed in Huysmans and Guibert's works – symptoms to be read politically from the outset? Is there not a risk of superimposing contemporary political issues on textual bodies that, through their own literary performativity, which moreover belongs to other eras, have no use for them?

A queer and phenomenological perspective, focused on the aesthetics of bodily symptomatic perceptions, will allow the crossing of three authors that should not "normally" meet, in a strictly contextualized, generic, historical, and political approach. The idea of the chapter is *to feel* the anachronical dimensions and the disorienting performativity of the *bodily* symptoms experienced by the characters in the literary texts, and to explore how the suffering bodies staged in the scenes escape the present of their experience, through their own embodied feelings and transformation into literary symbolism. By doing so, the chapter does not aim at becoming a piece of normative or ethical knowledge on Huysmans, Guibert, and Wojnarowicz, and even less so on syphilis, AIDS, and queer writings. It is not meant as an essay that would reconduct and crystallize them in their respective late centuries and critical contexts. Rather, the chapter hopes to become a *queer object* that would make the characters' sensitive *bodies* meet and dance together across their respective scenes. As Ahmed stresses in *Queer Phenomenology:*

> Queer objects support proximity between those who are supposed to live on parallel lines, *as points that should not meet*. A queer object hence makes contact possible. Or, to be more precise, a queer object would have a surface that supports such contact. The contact is bodily, and it unsettles that line that divides spaces as worlds, thereby creating other kinds of connections where unexpected things can happen. (169)

The writings of Huysmans, Guibert, and Wojnarowicz were, in fact, never compared in a bodily and queer way, thanks to the dominant propension of literature departments to artificially compartmentalize works in their geographical and historical context of creation and/or their genre. If the sensitive bodies, through their experience of queer moments, *lose* their "normal" place in space and time, therefore, it becomes capital not to bring them back to the place they "lost," but rather to embrace their "losses of place," their sensory failures, their feelings of disorientation. Queer moments of failure and disorientation are not only moments of reification, or even animalization of the suffering bodies, but also represent opportunities to *refigure* the bodies in space and time, to open and create new literary and artistic ways of being in the world. By embracing queer aesthetics, oblique sensations, and disorienting feelings, we can bridge unusual critical paths between different bodies and space-times that "normally" should not meet, as is the case with our authors – Huysmans, Guibert, and Wojnarowicz – and their respective *fin de siècle*.

I will analyze, throughout the chapter's sections, the materialization of various bodily symptoms – mainly hallucination, synesthesia, pain, and reminiscence of traumatic experiences – *felt* by the characters in the texts of Huysmans, Guibert, and Wojnarowicz. The neurotic visions and hallucinations of Jean Floressas des Esseintes, the misanthropic and implicitly syphilitic anti-hero of Huysmans's *Against the Grain*, in front of his monstrous flowers, as well as the scene in which a synesthesia caused by the creosote-like perfume of a whisky throws the aesthete's memories into the brutal reminiscence of his traumatic rotten tooth uprooting, will be compared to two scenes by Guibert and one scene from Wojnarowicz's writings. On Guibert's side, the analysis will explore the scene from his first AIDS writing where an "abscess appears on the back of [the narrator's] throat" (Guibert, *To the Friend* 52). Each painful swallowing throws Guibert's memories back in space and time to the dance floor of a Mexican dancehall, the Bombay, where an old whore "suddenly shoved her tongue down [his] throat like a crazed snake" (Guibert, *To the Friend* 52). The analysis will also explore the phenomenology and performativity of the scene in which, in his second AIDS writing, Guibert recalls his "first fibroscopy [that] had been a real nightmare" (Guibert, *Compassion Protocol* 45), a queer and traumatizing moment in which his body was brutally thrown in a disorienting and dehumanizing scene of "killing the pig down on the farm" (Guibert, *Compassion Protocol* 45). On Wojnarowicz's side, my analysis will explore the short story entitled "Memories that Smell Like Gasoline," in which the narrator's gaze falls on "that face" (Wojnarowicz 15) in a cinema hall: the gaze *on* and *from* that man's face throws the narrator's sensations into mind-blowing visions of bodily deformations and into the synesthetic reminiscence of the brutal rape he survived while hitch-hiking on a summer night, when he was a fifteen-year-old teenager, fifteen years earlier. The analysis will explore how the happenings of different symptoms, in the five scenes, turn the bodies at once into laboratories and actors of queer moments of disorientation, "when things do not stay in place" (Ahmed 170), but therefore can aesthetically re-symbolize through that loss of place.

## Feelings of Disorientation and the Aesthetics of Becoming an Object

In the chapter titled "Disorientation and Queer Objects" of her book *Queer Phenomenology*, Ahmed states:

> Disorientation as a bodily feeling can be unsettling, and it can shatter one's sense of confidence in the ground or one's belief that the ground on which we reside can support the actions that make a life feel livable. Such a feeling of shattering, or of being shattered, might persist, and become a crisis. Or the feeling itself might pass as the ground returns or as we return to the ground. (157)

Syntonizing the thought of phenomenologist James Aho, when he suggests in his work *The Things of the World: A Social Phenomenology*, that "every lifeworld is a coherency of things" (Aho II), Ahmed affirms in counterpoint that "queer moments happen when things fail to cohere," and that "in such moments of failure, when things do not stay in place or cohere as place, disorientation happens" (Ahmed 170). Queer moments are therefore to be understood as bodily feelings of disorientation that make bodies lose their "normal" place in space and time. However, those feelings are not without impact on the sensitive bodies' state. Following Ahmed, the collapsing of the "upright" body position in space and time, through its disorienting sensory failure, "is what causes the body ... to become an object alongside other objects. In simple terms, disorientation involves becoming an object" (Ahmed 159).

To precisely analyze those queer moments in the literary texts, an attention not only to the disorienting reification process suffered by the bodies needs to be sustained, "but also [to] the disorientation in how objects are gathered to create a ground, or to clear a space on the ground (the field)" (Ahmed 160). Those "fields," I will call them the "scenes" where the characters' bodies are at once disoriented and reified through their symptoms, therefore deploying "a queer aesthetic [that] is activated through the function of negation rather than in the mode of positivity" (Halberstam 110). Following Halberstam, "a particular form of darkness, a negativity really ..., can be called a queer aesthetic" (96). But darkness and negativity can also be creative. They can transform symptoms of pain and trauma into aesthetic motors of a queer symbolism that throw different sensations and space-times together. Therefore, I want to explore how symptoms staged in literary scenes can be approached as "constitutive instabilities" (Butler XIX) of embodied experiences of queer moments, able, through their aesthetic performativity, to transform feelings of failure and disorientation into "productive crisis" (Butler XIX).

Indeed, aesthetics are first and foremost a bodily, sensory, and sensitive assemblage of phenomena. Before 1821, when the term began to be defined as "of or pertaining to appreciation of the beautiful," the term was more broadly embracing its perceptual dimension. In fact, the term *aesthetic* dates from 1798, and is derived "from German Ästhetisch (mid-18c.) or French esthétique (which is from German), [and] ultimately from Greek aisthetikos [that means] 'of or for perception by the senses, perceptive,' of things" ("Aesthetic (n.)"). Therefore, aesthetics are not to be rationally confined in questions of taste, or in philosophical and ethical debates about what would be beautiful and what would be ugly. More generally, aesthetics need to embrace *every* phenomena that are "perceptible" and that, consequently, shape and affect bodies and worlds, whether it be in a good or bad way. Following its etymology, aesthetics can be understood not only through but *as* a bodily experience of sensations and feelings. Therefore, if "[queer] moments of disorientation ... are bodily experiences that throw the world up or throw the body from its ground" (Ahmed 157), their comprehension in literary texts needs to be addressed through their symptomatic aesthetics: the phenomenology of their feelings of disorientation in space and time, through the characters' senses (re)living the scenes, therefore opening creative possibilities of re-symbolization through failure.

## Huysmans and Des Esseintes

### *Entropic Performativity and Disorienting Symptoms of Syphilis*

In *Against the Grain*, the symptomatic aesthetics of syphilis manifests in multiple ways. In chapter VIII, in the scene in which flowers, each stranger than the next, are delivered to his estate in Fontenay, Des Esseintes observes:

> The men brought other and fresh varieties [of flowers], in this case presenting the appearance of a fictitious skin marked by an imitation network

> of veins. Most of them, as if disfigured by syphilis or leprosy, displayed livid patches of flesh, reddened by measles, roughened by eruptions; others showed the bright pink of a half-closed wound or the red brown of the crusts that form over a scar; others were as if scorched with cauteries blistered with burns; others again offered hairy surfaces eaten into holes by ulcers and excavated by chancres. (Huysmans, *Against the Grain* 85)

In Des Esseintes's neurotic eyes, syphilis does not only affect human bodies from the inside. Through the pantheist and protean performativity of his symptoms and visions, the so-called Great Pox emerges to the visible surface of nature and its objects, in a manner as novel as it is distorted. Syphilis symptoms *materialize* disfigurement processes in bodies, beings, and things, thus disorienting their representation in time and space, and the senses of those witnessing them. Under Huysmans' pen, the symptoms of syphilis give flesh to possibilities of mythical (re)symbolizing, while bringing together space-times that normally remain disjointed in a linear conception of history. His gaze hallucinated by the horde of sickly and monstrous flowers amassing in front of him, the neurotic aesthete muses:

> "It is all a matter of syphilis," reflected Des Esseintes, his eyes attracted, riveted on the hideous marking of the Caladiums, lit up at that moment by a shaft of daylight. And he had a sudden vision of the human race tortured by the virus of long past centuries. Ever since the beginning of the world, from sire to son, all living creatures were handing on the inexhaustible heritage, the everlasting malady that has devastated the ancestors of the men of to-day, has eaten to the very bone old fossil forms which we dig up at the present moment. (Huysmans, *Against the Grain* 89)

Although very phantasmagorical in style, Des Esseintes's reverie does not make of syphilis an ideal and metaphysical process, but rather one that is incarnate, visible, and organic, one that *materializes,* through the symptoms of disfigurement and disorientation, the (re)symbolizing potentialities through time and space, including through the sporadic emergence of survivals of "long past centuries" in the "present moment." "It's all a *matter* of syphilis" (I emphasize), astutely notes Havelock Ellis's English translation, given that the original French reads "Tout n'est que syphilis," which literally means "All is but syphilis." This perspective on the materiality of bodies and their power to (re)symbolize through symptoms can be inscribed in continuity to Judith Butler's 1993 *Bodies That Matter: On the Discursive Limits of "Sex,"* where the philosopher states:

> To speak within these classical contexts of bodies *that matter* is not an idle pun, for to be material means to materialize, where the principle of that materialization is precisely what matters about that body, its very intelligibility. In this sense, to know the significance of something is to know how and why it matters, where "to matter" means at once "to materialize" and "to mean." (Butler 7)

However, the signifying power of materiality is not to be taken as a static phenomenon, that would merely presume of the presence or the absence of a material entity – whether an object or a subject. Materiality is rather a dynamic phenomenon in time and space, whose symptoms, sensations, and perspectives drag along matter in *transformative* movements of its representations. As Ahmed rightly expresses: "It is crucial that 'matter' does not become an object that we presume is absent or present: what matters is shaped by the direction taken that allows things to appear in a certain way" (165). It is the movements and metamorphoses of matter – whether it is human, organic, vegetal, mineral, etc. – that provide it its relative and shifting appearance, from one embodied experience to the next. In a cult scene in *Against the Grain*, the mythical past of syphilis extracts itself from the present, first through the sickly symptoms that emerge "again" at the visible surface of the flowers, and second through the neurotic eyes of Des Esseintes, which perceive the flowers in an extraordinary manner: "Never wearying, [syphilis] had travelled down the ages, to this day it was raging everywhere, disguised under ordinary symptoms of headache or bronchitis, hysteria or gout; ... And lo! here it was reappearing, in its pristine splendor, on the bright-colored petals of flowers! (Huysmans, *Against the Grain* 89)

In Des Esseintes's famous musing, syphilis is therefore much more than a venereal disease specific to human beings. It becomes the aesthetic and symptomatic process that insufflates both vitality and morbidity to beings and to nature. Des Esseintes perceives syphilis as a drive of both life and death. It is a queer performative power of resistance to "normal" life, however not in the form of destruction, but rather through the deployment of (re)symbolizing that goes *against the grain* of sensory norms and of rigidly framed representational logics. In his essay *No Future: Queer Theory and the Death Drive*, published in 2004, Edelman explains that "queerness attains its ethical value precisely insofar as it accedes to that place, accepting its figural status as resistance to the viability of the social while insisting on the inextricability of such resistance from every social structure" (3). Resistance to viability – Edelman speaks of social viability, but we could very well transpose the argument to organic viability – would therefore be the principle of a "queer death drive" that would not be nihilistic but that would open potentialities by failing normalcy.

Under Huysmans' pen, syphilis thus appears to become the aesthetic and symptomatic principle of a "queer death drive" – which Edelman also designates as "sinthomosexuality" – that deviates bodies and things from their "normal" and "natural" course, at once organically, sensorially, and figuratively. Syphilis, as a "queer death drive," thus becomes an engine for sensation and (dis)figuration, against nature and, through a literary extension, against naturalism. In Des Esseintes's haywire eyes, as the illness works on him slyly, syphilis becomes, indeed, the aesthetic symptom of a death drive that destroys the boundaries separating human bodies from flowers, but also that disorients the sensations of the aesthete, whose sight errs into anachronic visions, runs aground against new configurations that knot together the symbolic, the imaginary and the real. According to Edelman, the symptom, or in the author's favoured spelling, the "sinthome" (in reference to Lacan), "speaks to the singularity of the subject's existence, to the particular way each subject manages to knot together the orders of the Symbolic, the Imaginary, and the Real" (Edelman 35). This triple knotting, however, could also be understood as a triple fall. The "etymology" of symptom, which means "fall together," allows us to clarify that the symptom is a happening in which the symbolic, the imaginary, and the real *fall*, and thus *fail*, together. It is the power of this "falling together" that makes (re)symbolizing possible, through the shock of the failures that the symptom materializes in bodies, sensations, and appearances.

*When Synesthesia Reactivates Traumatic Reminiscence*

Sensory and spatiotemporal disorientation is not limited to visual symptoms for Des Esseintes. It acts through *all* his senses, through symptoms pertaining to multiple sensations. Again in chapter VIII, Des Esseintes tastes a tiny cup of "genuine Irish whisky" (Huysmans, *Against the Grain* 46), whose strong flavour of creosote reactivates the traumatic memory of the brutal tooth extraction that he went through three years prior, while he was assailed with the most atrocious pain. The gustatory symptom concentrates the aesthete's scattered mind into a memorial tunnel that makes his thoughts converge onto a specific traumatic recollection: that of a treatment inflicted by "Gatonax," "a mechanic calling himself a dentist and living at the corner of a neighbouring street" (Huysmans, *Against the Grain* 47).

While Des Esseintes follows Gatonax into the "inner sanctum" (Huysmans, *Against the Grain* 47) of his house that serves as an operating room – his "field," could we say following Ahmed when she refers to the space where moments of queer disorientation occur – "his sensations had been vague" (Huysmans, *Against the Grain* 47) and "confusedly he remembered dropping into an armchair before a window, and stammering out, as he put a finger to his tooth: 'It has been stopped already; I am afraid there's nothing can be done'" (Huysmans, *Against the Grain* 48). However, Gatonax quickly interrupts Des Esseintes; he has no use for his explanations and sticks his huge finger into the patient's mouth, in search of the cause of his intolerable pain. Des Esseintes's sensory confusion is exacerbated by Gatonax's complete lack of interest for his suffering. It is from that moment – one of confusion, disorientation, and reification of the human body – that a queer scene unfolds, a queer *drama* to the extent that it makes Des Esseintes lose his mind and his head, provoking the crumbling of the soil under his feet. As we already saw, queer moments are "bodily experiences that throw the world up or throw the body from its ground" (Ahmed 157), and the disorientation they cause implicate "becoming an object" (Ahmed 159). That is what happens during the tooth extraction scene, during which the soil of the present gives way under Des Esseintes's feet, while his body in pain becomes but an object, a beast on the verge of being massacred.

> Thereupon the drama had begun. Clinging to the arms of the operating chair, Des Esseintes had felt a sensation of cold in his cheek, then his eyes had seen three dozen candles all at once, and so unspeakable were the tortures he was enduring, he had started beating the floor with his feet and bellowing like an animal under the slaughterer's knife. (Huysmans, *Against the Grain* 48)

His body's bestialization process is not only a metaphor; it is literal, materially embodied. It is Des Esseintes's corporeal sensations, combined with the treatment Gatonax inflicts on him, that transform him into a beast about to be slain. In that queer – and cruel – moment, bestialization is experimented through symptoms that disorient human sensation into inhuman symbols, lying out of humanity.

> There was a loud crack, the molar had broken in coming away; he thought they were pulling off his head, smashing in his skull; he lost all control of himself, howled at the top of his voice; fought furiously against the man who now came at him again as if he would plunge his arm to the bottom of his belly; had then suddenly stepped back a pace and lifting the patient bodily by the tooth still sticking in his jaw, had let him fall back again violently in a sitting posture into the chair; next moment he was standing

> up blocking the window, and puffing and panting as he brandished at the end of his pincers a blue tooth with a red thread hanging from it. (Huysmans, *Against the Grain* 48)

In this scene, Des Esseintes's body becomes fragmented. His embodied – and therefore aesthetic – experience gives him the clear impression of a decapitation and of an explosion of his skull. In the aftermath, Des Esseintes does not scream; he *bellows* and *howls* like a beast that Gatonax assaults to penetrate brutally to the depth of its entrails. At the apex of the scene, it seems that it is not the tooth that is extracted from the body, but rather the body that is torn off from the tooth, as it falls back on the operating chair like a lump of inert flesh. In trying to expunge the source of pain from Des Esseintes's human body, Gatonax pulls out all his humanity. This literary scene, even if it gives rise to a *fin de siècle* stylistic escalation, resonates in an anachronistic, even timeless, way with a criticism commonly formulated towards health systems: their dehumanization of the subjects they treat. Let us think, for example, of the words of Muzil/Foucault reported by Guibert, in his first AIDS narrative:

> Muzil spent a morning in the hospital having tests done, and told me he'd forgotten how completely the body loses all identity once it's delivered into medical hands, becoming just a package of helpless flesh, trundled around here and there, hardly even a number on a slip of paper, a name put through the administrative mill, drained of all individuality and dignity. (Guibert, *To the Friend* 23–24.)

To top things off, the "queer drama" lived by Des Esseintes, reactivated by the whisky synesthetic reminiscence, ends in a "darkness"– a dominant element of queer aesthetics according to Halberstam – that is as literary as it is literal: Gatonax obstructs the window of the operating "inner sanctum" and, hence, blocks with his imposing stature, reminding of that of an executioner, the light of day that would illuminate the scene. The queer drama is a scene of disorientation of the body into a sombre decor. It is the embodied drama of a becoming-object, a becoming-animal in a dark theatre of cruelty.

This queer moment of disorientation and bestialization comes to a – provisional – end with the relief of Des Esseintes's pain. As Ahmed explains, "Such a feeling of shattering, or of being shattered, might persist, and become a crisis. Or the feeling itself might pass as the ground returns or as we return to the ground" (157). Once his painful symptom is gone, Des Esseintes becomes again "a happy man, feeling ten years younger, ready to be interested in the veriest trifles" (Huysmans, *Against the Grain* 48). However, the queer moment of the rotten tooth uprooting does not vanish for good. Its potential for disorientation remains lurking, dormant in the aesthete's sensitive body. It may also resurface in the future, years later, when "dismal reminiscences" are reactivated by the synesthetic and anachronic tasting of Irish whisky, snug in the comfort of one's living room.

## Guibert

### *When Dancing Memories Erupt from under the Abscess*

In the first instalment of his AIDS trilogy, *To the Friend Who Did Not Save My Life*, Guibert keeps track of his body almost obsessively, in search for symptoms and signs that could lead him to believe he is HIV-positive. In 1983, "shortly after [his] return from Mexico, a huge abscess appeared on the back of [his] throat, which made swallowing difficult and eating impossible" (Guibert, *To the Friend* 32). For Guibert, not only are corporeal symptoms signs of disease, but they also become an integral part of his shifting relationship to time. Guibert's body is a calendar, and each symptom – whether his own or that of those around him – is a landmark event:

> 1983 was the year of Mexico, my throat abscess and Jules's swollen lymph nodes. 1984: Marine's and my editor's treachery toward me, Muzil's death, and the votive messages offered in Japan at the Temple of Moss. I don't find anything in 1985 relevant to our story. 1986 was the year the priest died. 1987 was my shingles. 1988 brought the revelation of my illness, a sentence without possibility of appeal, followed three months later by that chance event that managed to persuade me I could be saved. (Guibert, *To the Friend* 51)

In the eight years preceding the publication of his first AIDS writing, Guibert realized that "physiological accidents" are just as important as personal and sexual encounters in the relative unfolding of time. It is those accidents, those symptomatic happenings that regulate, or rather deregulate, his relationship to time. In Guibert's work, chronology is not strictly temporal: it is corporeal, embodied. Time is a sensation, and its dynamic is symptomatic.

> In this chronology summing up and pinpointing the warning signs of the disease over a period of eight years, when we now know that its incubation

> period is between four and a half and eight years, according to Stephane, the physiological accidents are no less decisive than the sexual encounters, the premonitions no less telling than the wishes that try to banish them. That's the chronology that becomes my outline, except whenever I discover that progression springs from disorder. (Guibert, *To the Friend* 51)

The unfolding of time, for Guibert, thus, is neither linear, nor regular, and especially, not predetermined. Its progression is paced either by physiological accidents – or even their premonition or anticipation – or by the disorder that becomes erected as a principle, at once corporeal and spatio-temporal. It is by disordering that the narration of the body, and that of its relationship to time, progresses. Guibert's progress, therefore, stops being a positive and positivist notion; on the contrary, it is a negative force, a drive that negates the order of things, that perturbates the normal balance of the body. While Ahmed states in *Queer Phenomenology* that "to make things queer is certainly to disturb the order of things" (161), Edelman writes, in *No Future*, that the queer "death drive marks the excess embedded within the Symbolic through the loss, the Real loss, that the advent of the signifier effects" (9). In that sense, Guibertian chronology appears to pertain to a queer death drive's aesthetic and symptomatic dynamic, as it is the perceptible occurrence of physiological accidents that move time ahead while also disordering it. In Guibert's works, time symbolizes through its loss of orientation, its disorder caused by his own or others' embodied symptoms.

Hence, "[when he gets] back from Mexico in October of 1983 and this abscess appears on the back of [his] throat, [Guibert doesn't] know which doctor to turn to" (Guibert, *To the Friend* 52). He is distraught, disoriented, desperate. Each swallow is painful, and the abscess leads Guibert in a process of reminiscence that reactivates the memory of a crazy evening in a Mexican dancehall. The symptom becomes an aesthetic source of spatiotemporal disorientation, an organic time travel machine: "With this white, raw wound festering on my throat, I'm haunted by the kiss I got in Mexico on the dance floor of the Bombay from the old whore who ... had suddenly shoved her tongue down my throat like a crazed snake" (Guibert, *To the Friend* 53). Through the pain it causes, and as the gustatory synesthesia caused by the strong scent of creosote did for Des Esseintes, Guibert's abscess becomes a symptomatic passage between bodies and space-times. Guibert's body communicates from his Paris apartment with the body of the prostitute who forcibly kissed him in Mexico during his recent trip there: "The old whore had crossed the line ...: without warning she'd stuck her tongue down my throat, and thousands of kilometers away, each twinge of pain from my abscess brought back her kiss, which dug ever deeper into the sore like the tip of a white-hot branding iron (Guibert, *To the Friend* 53). Like his body wracked with pain, Guibert's writing is carried away in an aesthetic whirlpool where sensations and space-times dance together. In *Queer Phenomenology*, Ahmed writes: "What is so compelling to me about this account of 'becoming queer' is how the strangeness that seems to reside somewhere between the body and its objects is also what brings these objects to life and makes them dance" (163). In this scene, Guibert's body seems to become queer through his painful symptom, since it is its unexpected occurrence that disorients his sensations and make space-times dance together. In the frensy of his painful reminiscence, Guibert lives anew – and transcribes through the same movement – a furious scene in which a horde of prostitutes dance around him, and turn his body into a blonde idol. Guibert's body, through the dance of the memories caused by his abscess, reifies into a cult-worthy fetish that attracts envy and disorder around it.

The Bombay dancehall is not the only place Guibert visits during his Mexican travel. When he goes "to a homosexual nightclub at the urging of Jules's Mexican friend, ... the boys had lined up in front of [him] in the same way to stare and the bolder ones had reached out to touch [him] as though [he was] a lucky charm" (Guibert, *To the Friend* 53). Such reification of Guibert's body into a "lucky charm" is reactivated by the painful abscess that's opening deep in his throat. The symptom, by breaking his physical integrity, also interrupts his temporal linearity: it activates a process in which the sensation of disorientation reifies bodies and make space-times collide.

### *"Killing the Pig down on the Farm": Obscene Bodies and Queer Space-Time*

While the reminiscence caused by the strong creosote perfume revived, on Des Esseintes' tongue, Gatonax's brutal tooth extraction that turned him, for the time of a "drama," in a beast fit for the slaughterhouse, in Guibert's work, it is the traumatizing recollection of a fibroscopy that engraves itself in his memory. Guibert tells that grotesque and bestializing event, which he qualifies as torture, in the second instalment of his AIDS trilogy: "The first fibroscopy had been a real nightmare: killing the pig down on the farm. The Rothschild Hospital, Professor Bihiou's gastro-enterology service, torture chambers on the ground floor" (Guibert, *Compassion Protocol* 45). While Des Esseintes's drama began with Gatonax rushing at him in grenadier garb to tear out his tooth in such a brutal manner that the aesthete felt he became "an animal under the slaughterer's knife" (Huysmans, *Against the Grain* 48) Guibert's scene, for its part, begins with the sensational arrival of a "commando of torturers" that transform him into a beast to be impaled alive:

> At once the door bursts open, and the commando of torturers rushes in and throws itself upon me. ... a distracted student nurse, to whom Dr Domer, a grimace of disgust on his face, is issuing orders from a safe distance, stuffs this thick tube into my mouth and forces it past my uvula so as to shove it down inside me. I'm suffocating, I cannot take this tube they are thrusting down my trachea until it reaches my stomach, I have spasms, contractions, hiccups, I want to reject it, spit it out, vomit it out of me, I am slavering and groaning. The thought of suicide comes back, of the most absolute form of physical humiliation, the most definitive. (Guibert, *Compassion Protocol* 46)

Whereas in the previous sections, it was Gatonax's arm that was plunged to the bottom of Des Esseintes's belly, and the Mexican prostitute's "crazed snake" tongue that was shoved into Guibert's throat, in the fibroscopy scene, it is a "thick tube" that is forced down and wounds his trachea. The tube marks Guibert's throat with a trauma that – like the white abscess that appeared in his throat when he returned from Mexico – will reopen again in the future, not from synesthesia, but from the act of writing. However, and like the symptomatic synesthesia in *Against the Grain*, where the creosote taste reoccurs years later, in Guibert it is not instantly "translatable" into literary language. While Des Esseintes forgets his experience as soon as it ends and his pain fades, only to surge again years later, in Guibert the trauma of the fibroscopy is such that he is unable, when he is back home, to align two words in his diary to write about it.

> When I got home, I opened my journal and wrote: "Fibroscopy." Nothing else, nothing more, no explanation, no description of the examination and no commentary on my sufferings, it was impossible to put two words together, I was speechless, mouth agape. I had become incapable of recounting my experience. (Guibert, *Compassion Protocol* 47)

The symptoms of pain, of disorientation, and of reification are so brutal, at that moment, that they destroy Guibert's language. In her famous book *The Body in Pain: The Making and Unmaking of the World*, published in 1985, Elaine Scarry states that "physical pain does not simply resist language but actively destroys it, bringing about an immediate reversion to a state anterior to language, to the sounds and cries a human being makes before language is learned" (4). Symptoms experienced during the fibroscopy leave Guibert speechless, and it is only much later that the fibroscopy's "queer moment" – queer in Ahmed's sense that it reifies his body, in addition to disorienting him, even expelling him from space-time of the present – will become, for Guibert's body, *signifying* and transcribable into novel writing.

During the procedure, the pain becomes at one point so unbearable that Guibert tears out the black tube shoved down his throat, only for it to be pushed back in by the intern under Domer's orders, "forcing it inside [him] until it reached the pit of [his] stomach" (Guibert, *Compassion Protocol* 47). At that time, Guibert "was trying to concentrate so as not to eject it again" (Guibert, *Compassion Protocol* 47). Suffocating, desperate, at the mercy of the "commando of pig-stickers" (Guibert, *Compassion Protocol* 47), Guibert's body is kept afar not only in physical distance but also spatio-temporally. Dr Domer considers Guibert as "nothing more than just another infected little faggot, who [is] going to kick the bucket in any case": he considers his suffering body not only as "wasted time" but also as undifferentiated – and possibly inhuman – material to be kept *at a distance*. "Dr Domer ... looked through the eyepiece, *still from a distance* [I emphasize], and said: 'There is an oesophagial candidiasis, quite definitely, one can diagnose it with the naked eye, and there are two ulcerations in the stomach, we must do the biopsies'" (Guibert, *Compassion Protocol* 47).

Even though the painful symptoms disappear following the brutal procedure, as was the case when Gatonax extracted Des Esseintes's tooth, Guibert knows very well that it traumatized him and that it would leave marks that would reopen in the future: "It was all over, I no longer felt pain, I could now tell myself it was all behind me, but I knew very well how this examination, performed in such a manner, must have traumatized me" (Guibert, *Compassion Protocol* 48). Unlike Des Esseintes though, who would marvel at the smallest things on leaving Gatonax's place, Guibert knows that his symptoms are only on borrowed time, in temporary dormancy. For, although his bestializing in the hands of the commando is over, Guibert anticipates that his painful, confusing and humiliating symptoms will resurface in the future. Perhaps not in the immediate future of the fibroscopy, but in a remote future, when Guibert would be able to take the pen to revive the experience for the time of his novel writing.

## Wojnarowicz

### *Resurging Trauma from a Disembodied and Floating Face*

"It's that face. I knew I'd seen it before" (Wojnarowicz 15). In the eponymous text of the collection *Memories That Smell Like Gasoline*, published in 1992, Wojnarowicz tells his chance and abrupt encounter with a face "in the lobby of a movie theater surrounded by crowds of people waiting to enter the auditorium" (15). In the chaotic confusion between two movie projections, while the "the doors flung open and hundreds of people were pouring out towards the exits" (Wojnarowicz 15), the narrator sees, among the bodies rushing towards the exit, a face that first appears anonymous, but whose vision gradually becomes distorted, taking him into a reminiscence that is as hallucinating as it is nightmarish.

> Suddenly that face. It was one anonymous face in the crowd that tripped the switch in the back of my head. I froze and the face became magnified. It expanded in size until it was five feet tall and disembodied and floating in the darkness of the open doors. I guess he froze too. He was a pale gray color with fastidiously combed hair plastered down around the skull. Thin lips, bloodless and tight. His eyes were colorless and they widened for a moment. We stood there trying to uncoil each other's private histories and solve the dislocation of familiarity. (Wojnarowicz 15)

From the onset of the scene, the "dislocation of familiarity" takes place through the perceptual symptoms embodied in the narrator. The magnification of the anonymous face takes gigantic, monstruous proportions in the narrator's vision. The moment's familiarity is dislocated at the same time as the anonymous head dislocates from the body that carries it. Through the movie theatre's lobby, and the darkness – a capital component of queer aesthetics – that pours in through the open doors, the head expands, floats in air in a bewildering manner, while the two protagonists – the narrator and the anonymous man – review their mutual stories, in search of the one that might connect them. From the start of "Memories that Smell Like Gasoline," it is the narrator's symptomatology, triggered by the expansive deformation of the floating face and the darkness of the decor, that disorients him both sensorily and spatiotemporally.

Progressively, a bodily recollection starts forming in the narrator's memory: "That face. When I noticed his suit and his hands, palms back and manicured nails, I remembered. Maybe it was the quality of light or lack of it in the lobby.... Maybe it was the colour of his flesh, the look of no oxygen, the look of anticipation or fear, the complexion of anticipation" (Wojnarowicz 16). The visions of the gigantic floating head, and the other physical particularities of the man's body, transport Wojnarowicz to the past, to the summer when he was fifteen and "a kid prostitute in New York City" (Wojnarowicz 15). That summer, he had taken a bus to escape from the city for a day, in the countryside, to wade in a pond. After his swim, the narrator hitchhikes his way back to NYC, and that is when the grey head appears for the first time to him, floating and dislocated, as it will appear to him fifteen years later, in the theatre lobby:

> Those eyes, that face gray and floating disembodied in the dark of the open window. A small beat-up red pick-up truck coasted to a stop along the side of the road. He was waving me into the truck. I remember thinking his skin was fake, like a semi-translucent latex. I asked him how far he was going. "Oh, a ways." (Wojnarowicz 17)

Wojnarowicz then boards the vehicle, which drives for a few moments in dark countryside, while the driver pulls his penis out of his pants and begins to masturbate. After a while, the truck turns off to the left on a small gravel road and goes deep into a forest, before stopping in a small clearing. After refusing to fellate him, the narrator is grabbed by the grey-face and latex-skinned man, who then opens the back door of the pick-up truck, throwing him into its moist and suffocating darkness, like in a living nightmare.

> One of his hands floated up to my face and then encircled the back of my neck and I realized I was being propelled forward towards the black interior of the camper. I crawled obediently inside, it was loaded with blankets and sleeping bags and boxes of indecipherable stuff. It was kind of moist and smelled like earth and grease. He climbed in behind me and pulled the door shut. Everything was reduced to smells and the sound of trees and the squeak of his shoes against the metal parts of the floor. I lay down and curled up on a mass of smelly cloth. I could see his silhouette half-rise before me, blocking out the minimal light and then dropping to my side. The sound of a zipper opening. His hand on my neck again. Pulling. I want to go home, I said. (Wojnarowicz 20)

Wojnarowicz is forcibly pushed into the darkness created by the combined effects of the night, of the indecipherable character of the "stuff" that litters the vehicle's floor, and of the imposing stature of his assailant who blocks the little light shining at that time, like Gatonax was blocking the window at the end of Des Esseintes's drama. In addition, the place teems with suffocating sensations – the unpleasant and damp smell of soil, grease, and clothes, the rattle of the trees among that of the assailant's shoes knocking the metallic tools strewn around. Wojnarowicz's body is dragged into a nightmarish moment during which he is turned into an object. He is also propelled into a sensory disorientation in which the missing light is replaced with an overload of scents and noises. The disorientation is also spatio-temporal, as the inside of the vehicle, littered with "indecipherable stuff," seems lost in the darkness of a countryside summer night.

"I couldn't see anything. The rain was coming down hard; sheets of water making the dimness more dark.... You like it in your ass? No. Good, he said and then hit me. Very hard" (Wojnarowicz 21). The narrator then describes the assault through a writing that is highly sensory and disturbing, where his body turns into an indistinct mass of flesh that literally loses sight of the world around: "I'm blind to the world and he's turning me over and over and over. Where am I?" (Wojnarowicz 21). In his assailant's stranglehold of violence, the narrator feels thrown into the night like an object, at the same time as his hands are tied behind his back with a pale rope: "I feel like I'm in motion like something flung out of a giant sling shot" (Wojnarowicz 21). Emotion, like the motion of Wojnarowicz's tied up and beaten body, is one of sensory and spatio-temporal disorientation that, at the same time, reifies it. That queer moment feels like an eternity to the narrator – "Funny how everything all my life moved excruciatingly slow until this moment and now I'm just begging for it to stop" (Wojnarowicz 24). During that time, he sees his assailant's head floating grotesquely in the dark interior of the pick-up truck, as if it were detached from his body – "He's pulling my hair, yanking my head back so his face appears upside down floating before mine and he's smiling. But the smile looks like a frown, it's upside down and he leans in and kisses both my eyes" (Wojnarowicz 23). The floating head forces the narrator to close his eyes by kissing them, and then he assaults him brutally. During the explicit and confusing aggression, Wojnarowicz's becomes his assailant's possession – "He treats me like he owns me" (Wojnarowicz 24) – as he is turned and returned in all directions: "Turning over and over and over what the fuck is he doing that for?" (Wojnarowicz 24).

In the chaos of the pick-up that's overloaded with violence, smells, and noises, soaked into the moist and musky darkness where his torturer's head floats upside down, the narrator hears his assailant commit a manoeuvre that exacerbates – as if it were possible – the scene's brutality.

> He lunges and reaches far into the darkness of the truck and I hear a container of liquid, sounds like a metal container and liquid sounds the image of lighter fluid or gasoline went through my mind. Is this it? I could see the flames; I could see my body being turned over by campers looking like a side of beef left too long in the fire, black and charred with bones

> poking out of it. I felt a squirt of liquid all over my ass, a memory smell from my childhood flooding the truck. Baby oil. I just want to die, I just want to die, I just want to die.... I'm sinking in dark pools of atmosphere. (Wojnarowicz 24–25)

Wojnarowicz's memory, at the sight of the floating head in the theater lobby, ends with his assailant forcibly sodomizing him, after having coated his butt cheeks with an uncertain liquid – gasoline or baby oil? In the traumatic scene, although the liquid *sounds* like the *image* of gasoline, it *smells* like baby oil. In the wake of such disorientation, where sounds, images, and smells clash, Wojnarowicz imagines himself burning like a savagely killed and carbonized beast, in the night, submerged not so much with "memories that smell like gasoline," but with "memories that smell like baby oil."

### *"Something Weird Happens": Falling out of Shape, Language, and Space-Time*

Reminiscing is, for Wojnarowicz, a common process, during which his personal stories, depending on specific sensory and spatio-temporal circumstances, can either escape him and disappear or dash towards him, like a floating head, to envelop him with synesthetic memories that are embodied, sensitive, and that may, at any time, shift into a nightmare:

> In the codes that I carry in the sleepy part of my head, personal histories can turn on a dime and either rush away into disintegration or else turn and speed towards me looking to envelop. In the moment he was swept up in the crowd and moving across the lobby toward me I shrunk mentally and in size like a kid with no defense not even my pocket knife.... It was like he was bleeding me right there in the crowded room. All my history and language had suddenly been erased. (Wojnarowicz 25–26)

Not only is Wojnarowicz's body affected by the sight of the "floating head" approaching him, from the darkness of his past assault, it is also both mentally and physically transformed, shrunk into his fifteen years old defenseless and suffering body: "I was stuck looking at him through the eyes of a fifteen-year-old skull.... Something weird happened where I physically shrunk and I took the moment where he and I lost track of each other to duck down the staircase to restrooms" (Wojnarowicz 26).

It is the symptomatic vision of the floating head that makes Wojnarowicz's body fall out of his present shape, language, and space-time. The reminiscence of his trauma is therefore not an abstract re-symbolization of the event through language, but an embodied and anachronistic revival of the symptoms that scared, and scarred, the body, and that are reactivated through the sensitive dislocation of familiarity that opens the scene. This "weird happening" will, however, linger after the man and his floating head are gone, along with the sounds, visions, and smells of that creepy night: "When I finally went back upstairs he seemed gone. But I could still feel his gaze; it lingered like the stink after a bad fire" (Wojnarowicz 26).

## Bodies that *Obliquely* Matter: From Bodily Symptoms to Queer Literary Symbolism

According to Butler, the body's materiality is attributable to its "performativity" – "[which] must be understood ... as the reiterative and citational practice by which discourse produces the effects that it names" (XII). This performativity must be continuously done over again, with the ever-present possibility of being deformed or deviated in alterities, rather than being safely crystalized in normativity and familiarity. Butler explains that "[bodily] materialization is never quite complete, that bodies never quite comply with norms by which their materialization is impelled," and that "it is the instabilities, the possibilities of rematerialization, opened up by this process that mark one domain in which the force of the regulatory law can be turned against itself to spawn rearticulations that call into question the hegemonic force of that very regulatory law" (XII).

The chapter explored, through different embodied experiences of queer moments – sometimes utterly cruel and traumatizing – how symptoms can aesthetically disorient, reify, or even animalize sensitive bodies. Des Esseintes was able to feel the untimely performativity of the Great Pox through the diseased *materiality* of his flowers, and his hypersensitive body was also thrown back in time towards the uprooting of a rotten tooth, a reminiscence that was performatively actualized by a creosote-like taste in his mouth. A similar process seemed at work on Guibert's side, when the pain caused by his unexpected abscess propelled him into a reminiscence of frantic dances in Mexico, where he would be reified in a "lucky charm," touched, and forcibly kissed, even "shoved," by the "crazed snake" tongue of an old dancing prostitute. Guibert's body was also brutally disoriented, reified, and marked by the nightmarish fibroscopy he underwent at Rothschild Hospital, in a way similar to how Wojnarowicz's body was marked by the assault he experienced as a fifteen-year-old. Even if the scenes analyzed in the chapter are from different authors, genres, and times, their comparison offers a queer perspective that cuts across their aesthetic particularities and that puts the sensitive and material symptoms *of the bodies* back in the spotlight, even though it is through dark scenes. In *No Future*, Edelman conceives of the performativity of the "sinthome" in those terms:

> Though it functions as the necessary condition for the subject's engagement of Symbolic reality, the sinthome refuses the Symbolic logic that determines the exchange of signifiers; it admits no translation of its singularity and therefore carries nothing of meaning, recalling in this the letter as the site at which meaning comes undone. (35)

Throughout the literary analysis conducted in this chapter, I wanted to shed light on the different ways in which symptoms refuse the symbolic logic of normal bodies, which deploys a linear conception of time. I wanted to explore how symptoms not only emerge when "meaning comes undone," as Edelman states, but also how meaning can flourish anew, in an oblique way, from its very material failures. Stated otherwise, this chapter has sought to elucidate how bodies can *obliquely* matter through other space-times than the ones of their experiences. In *The Queer Art of Failure*, Halberstam conceptualizes this form of "art" following Walter Benjamin, whose "relation to knowing [is] a stroll down uncharted streets in the 'wrong' direction" (Halberstam 6), as opposed to "staying in well-lit territories and about knowing exactly which way to go before you set out" (Halberstam 6). This is what the chapter hopes to have accomplished: lose its way by embracing Huysmans, Guibert, and Wojnarowicz's queer, dark, but also untimely aesthetics.

## WORKS CITED

Ahmed, Sara. *Queer Phenomenology: Orientations, Objects, Others*. Duke UP, 2006.

Aho, James A. *The Things of the World: A Social Phenomenology*. Praeger, 1998.

Butler, Judith. *Bodies That Matter: On the Discursive Limits of "Sex."* 1993. Routledge, 2011.

Edelman, Lee. *No Future: Queer Theory and the Death Drive*. Duke UP, 2004.

Guibert, Hervé. *L'image Fantôme*. Editions de Minuit, 1981.

–. *To the Friend Who Did Not Save My Life*. Translated by Linda Coverdale, Quartet, 1991.

–. *Compassion Protocol*. Translated by James Kirkup, Quartet Books, 1995.

Halberstam, Judith. *The Queer Art of Failure*. Duke UP, 2013.

Huysmans, Joris-Karl. *Against the Grain (À Rebours)*. Translated by Havelock Ellis, Dover Publications, 1969. *Internet Archive*, http://archive.org/details/againstgrainareb00huys.

–. *À Rebours*. 1884. Edited by Marc Fumaroli, Gallimard, 1999.
Rancière, Jacques. *The Politics of Aesthetics: The Distribution of the Sensible*. Edited by Gabriel Rockhill, Bloomsbury Revelations edition, Bloomsbury Academic, 2013.
Scarry, Elaine. *The Body in Pain: The Making and Unmaking of the World*. Oxford UP, 1985.
Wojnarowicz, David. *Memories that Smell Like Gasoline*. Artspace, 1992.

# 6 Positive Status/Positive Space: The Opportunity of Disclosure

ERIC JORGENSEN

While leading a seminar for upper-division undergraduate theatre students on the American AIDS plays, I became haunted and angered by an article: "Brilliant, 41 and Lost to AIDS: The Theater World Asks Why" (Paulson). It appeared in the theatre section of the *New York Times* – partly an obituary, partly an indictment of the theatre community for neglecting one of their own. A young, talented musical theatre composer-lyricist, entering his prime, poised to be one of the greats, died of AIDS. The article documents his last few months as he furiously struggled to meet deadlines. He had stacks of projects with different collaborators in various states of incompletion. There was the recent out-of-town opening of his new show that he was never able to attend and the resourceful ways he would deliver score rewrites to the production's musical director while attached to a ventilator in a hospital ward. Giants of the theatre world recalled seeing him wasting away over the last few months of his life. They noticed strange purple lesions on his face and a missing fire behind his eyes, but they were reluctant to invade the privacy of someone they knew as an exuberant but fiercely private man. The once-buoyant soul could barely ascend a flight of stairs without support, and the assumption of those around him was that he was ill but would soon be better. This might be the story of so many theatre artists who died of AIDS in the worst days of the plague. But what is maddening about this particular panegyric is not the familiar story, but rather the date of its publication – October 15, 2017.

I cannot say that I knew Michael Friedman. We had a few shared friends, and I auditioned for him at least once, but our paths never crossed beyond that. I admired his work. His musical adaption of *Love's Labour's Lost* that graced the summer season at Central Park's Delacorte Theater in 2013 dusted off Shakespeare's most frivolous work and made it completely contemporary. His musical *Bloody, Bloody, Andrew*

*Jackson* was something of a precursor to *Hamilton* in that it proved written biographies of American historical figures as viable source material for musical theatre. That is likely where the comparison should leave off, as the tone of the two musicals could not be more dissimilar. But like *Hamilton*, *Bloody, Bloody* was a bona fide hit in its original Off-Broadway incarnation, and its recognition rocketed its composer-lyricist to the top of the New York theatre's unofficial list of people to watch.

There are at least two notable ways in which Michael's work figures into the corpus of American AIDS drama. In 2010, Signature Theatre Company produced the first major New York City revival of both parts of Kushner's *Angels in America.* With a starry cast in a jewel box of a theatre, the anticipation was palpable, and ticket buyers lined up more than two days before the box office opened. The limited Off-Broadway run sold out in minutes. Michael composed an original musical score to accompany the seven-hour play. Also among the projects left unfinished at the time of his death was a sequel to the quintessential American musical about the American musical, *A Chorus Line.* Whereas the original musical about a group of auditioning dancers is set in 1975, the continuation that Michael was pursuing with several close collaborators would have been set a decade later, as that same generation of dreamers was ravaged by AIDS.

The unprecedentedly long original run of *A Chorus Line* is itself a case study in how plays not about AIDS become threaded into the fabric of the AIDS drama corpus. It was precisely at the midpoint of *A Chorus Line*'s fifteen-year run when AIDS became known. Almost immediately, there were multiple AIDS deaths among the ranks of Broadway singers and dancers. The gritty sparkle of *A Chorus Line*, in which the characters sing and dance of sacrifice and survival, and in which they promise that they "won't forget, can't regret" giving their all for the love of their art, suddenly seemed anachronistic without mention of the plague that was robbing that very art of some of its most loving souls. At the same time, the setting in a time before AIDS may well have been a haven for those needing a matinee escape from the harsh daily reminders of the plague. Three of *A Chorus Line's* five creators: director-choreographer Michael Bennett and book writers James Kirkwood, Jr. and Nicholas Dante, would die of AIDS before the show ended its original Broadway run. So AIDS is absent in the world of the text but indelibly present in the worlds of the audience and the playwright.

In Larry Kramer's 2014 screenplay adaptation of his 1985 play *The Normal Heart*, one man – a minor character in the play, a major character in the film – stands to eulogize another young man. He speaks of how funerals and memorials have become the social life of the time.

He speaks of his own anger and how it seems that nobody is offering to help. Then he offers another thought, "We're losing an entire generation. Young men at the beginning, just gone. Choreographers, playwrights, dancers, actors. All those plays that won't get written now. All those dances never to be danced." This line is not spoken in the play, and its utterance in the film signals the distance traveled in the twenty-nine years between the two scripts. There was no time for sentimentality in 1985, when remembrance needed to be secondary to rage – a particular rage that galvanized a diminishing population. But three decades later, this line informs a different story. Melancholia, both primary and acquired, is a powerful state that provides space to consider what we lost, or in this case, what never was.

If Michael Friedman and his collaborators were to have completed their sequel project, perhaps conceived as *A Chorus Line 2: The Wrath of AIDS*, the AIDS musical might very well be the nexus for AIDS nostalgia, fear, and melancholia. One can only speculate how this musical might have been received. Rage and sentimentality doubtlessly would have shaped the narrative. Michael's death from AIDS more than thirty years after the time in which the sequel to *A Chorus Line* was to have been set makes the metanarrative of the musical powerfully prescient. The impetus for the project was the unending need to redefine survival – art, creation in the face of death, hope springing from cynicism. But Michael's death likewise resonates with Kramer's sentimental departure. Kramer left out composers from his list of professions where unique voices were being snuffed out one by one. It is thoroughly disquieting in the midst of AIDS cultural reticence and complacency that Kramer's line rings clear and present. Michael Friedman, a young man at the beginning, just gone. All those musicals that won't get written now.

Equally unnerving in the *New York Times* finger-pointing article about Michael's death are the voices that should have known better; this, at least if one considers the theatre as a place where knowledge is transferred. Michael had health insurance as an employee of the Public Theater. He was officially listed as Director of Public Forum and Artist in Residence, but he was universally recognized as a creative force and an ideal collaborator. Oskar Eustis, The Public's artistic director, is quoted in the article remarking that this was "a real warning shot across the bow for anybody who thinks this disease isn't deadly anymore. It just killed one of the most brilliant and promising people in the American theater" (Paulson). Director Michael Greif is quoted as saying, "I wish I could have done more. I wish I had known more. I wish I could have interceded more. I wish that I could have found a way to let Michael let me be a better friend to him, and I regret that I wasn't able to do that"

(Paulson). Indeed. Michael reported for work daily to the very theatre where the first mainstream American play about AIDS, *The Normal Heart*, premiered and extended to a record-breaking Public Theater run. Eustis is largely responsible for commissioning Tony Kushner's *Angels in America*, and he directed its premiere at The Mark Taper Forum in Los Angeles. Eustis also was the director of Paula Vogel's second major AIDS play, *The Long Christmas Ride Home*. Greif is perhaps best known in musical theatre circles as the original director of *Rent*, the most commercially successful AIDS play ever. And it was while directing Signature Theatre's revival production of *Angels in America* that he first worked with Michael. These two directors seemingly knew Michael as well as any professional colleague did. They are among the most significant figures in American AIDS theatre. I contend that the American stage provided the location for one of the most significant understandings of the pandemic. How is it possible that Michael could have been in the most severe and final phases of HIV disease and these colleagues, these particular colleagues, either did not notice or did not intervene? Have the American AIDS plays and their caretakers become so contentedly secure in believing AIDS to be a thing of the past, that a "warning shot" is suddenly necessary? Conveniently, theatre artists have at their disposal thirty-five years' worth of plays ready to teach them about not only the history of the pandemic but also about how AIDS crystalized a need for interconnectedness and human compassion.

Yet no one is to blame.

Susan Sontag wrote, "It seems that societies need to have one illness which becomes identified with evil, and attaches blame to its "victims," but it is hard to be obsessed with more than one" (*Illness as Metaphor* 104) According to *The New York Times* article (Paulson), when Michael died on September 9, it was just nine weeks after his doctor told him that he had tested positive for HIV. While the immediate course of antiretrovirals began its lengthy process of stopping his virus in its various stages of replication, the medical options for his advanced and compounding illnesses quickly ran out. His immune system was gone. In those nine weeks, Michael was first hospitalized for ten days and then sent home when marginal improvement showed a suggestion of recuperation. Three weeks before his death, Michael was readmitted to the hospital with acute respiratory distress syndrome. He spent the rest of his life in intensive care, intubated and sedated. The consensus among those close to him is that Michael waited too long to seek medical attention. While there are known cases of rapid AIDS progression, the incubation period between acute HIV infection and what was once called full-blown AIDS is typically several years. Eustis said, "As near as I can tell, he hadn't actually been to a doctor or gotten tested for a couple of years, and only in July did he find out that he was HIV positive. That's just staggering – staggeringly wrong of Michael, staggeringly upsetting" (Paulson).

The article goes on to describe the memorial service that followed one week after his death. With New York theatre luminaries among the several hundred friends in attendance, Michael was remembered for his work, for his indomitable spirit, and for his humour. At one point between the silences involved in the Quaker service, playwright Eisa Davis posed a question, "I just wonder if Michael loved himself as much as we loved him?" (Paulson). In the wake of his death and because of its cause, those closest to Michael questioned his assessment of his self-worth. But how deeply does this questioning bore? If Michael had loved himself more, then he would have sought medical treatment earlier. But he didn't know he was dying. If he had loved himself more, then he would have been tested for HIV years earlier. The Centers for Disease Control estimate that one in five Americans with HIV is unaware of their status. If Michael Friedman had loved himself more, then he wouldn't have put himself at risk for HIV. This is the exact moralizing that was fought compassionately by playwrights, actors, and characters throughout decades of American AIDS plays. Full circle, those who led the fight on the theatrical front are now chinning the victims.

The risk in cultural incorporation of HIV/AIDS is its relegation to another time or place. In turn, AIDS becomes an abstraction, something not here and now, but then and there. Thus, the consequence for how one should teach this topic involves a de-abstraction of HIV/AIDS. In order to fully convey the various ways in which the corpus of AIDS dramatic material represents the evolution of the pandemic, it is of utmost importance to introduce the material as something that relates to the here and now. It is here that disclosure of my own status might make my point clear. I do not view my HIV status as something I need to keep secret; my caveat, however, is that it is a piece of information that I alone control when to share. Others have remarked that in bringing my serostatus to my work, and, frankly, in conjoining it with a lifelong passion for the theatre, that I have somehow done something brave. I say it is non traditionally academic, perhaps, but not a matter of bravery. Shame and pride regarding my HIV status have long ago dissolved or buried themselves in some forgotten place. But unpacking the language of those who declare that public disclosure is something akin to an act of bravery, it is implied that disclosure is an act worthy of remark. In a sense, disclosure is an Austinian performative utterance. What once was unknown cannot ever again not be known. Therefore, the speaking of a word has changed the condition, not for me, the person living with

HIV, but rather for the others for whom this is a new piece of information. The remarkable thing about the act of disclosure then is not that I have broken some sort of expected silence, but rather that it brings out the issue of why that silence might be expected in the first place. Certainly, in the case of HIV, a pervasive social stigma remains.

The single most important thing I am able to do to fight HIV stigma is to disclose my status. In doing so, at least for that moment, HIV/AIDS ceases to be an abstraction. It is no longer something that devastatingly did happen at one time, nor is it something that can be geographically distanced by the separation of an ocean. When I inform an individual or a group that I am HIV-positive, the virus cannot merely be a clinically studied pathogen. AIDS is not a day of red-ribbon remembrance or a quilt of commemoration. HIV is suddenly something other than an idea to be prevented or guarded against. In speaking the words, HIV is present and embodied. To repurpose Martin Buber's words, in disclosing, I body forth.

Disclosure in this context is likewise a vital teaching element. In addressing the entire corpus of American AIDS drama, it is important to lean into that which makes the theatre an irreplaceable medium. Theatre is live; drama is living. In embodying characters on stage who live with or deal directly with HIV/AIDS, actors and the plays in which they are performing send the disease through a process of de-abstraction. In the world of the audience, within the shared space of the theatre, audiences are confronted by the living presence of HIV/AIDS. In a real sense, this is the same confrontation that is brought about by face-to-face disclosure. In disclosing my status to others, I implicitly raise the question of why disclosure is itself significant. In sharing the space with characters living with AIDS, audiences must confront the reason why HIV/AIDS status is made a defining character trait or a central element of the play. They do so with their own cultural understanding of AIDS borne out of contemporary medical, global, and social reality. At least momentarily, the living presence on stage is the catalyst for this present-day transformation of AIDS from abstract concept to a tangible and energetic presence. So too is drama a living document; it is reinvented with each production and every audience; AIDS is at least revisited with renewed perspective. As disclosure is a performative act that raises the question of serostatus remarkability, live theater is the event that demands a confrontation with AIDS abstraction by making it physically present.

The act of disclosure has been compared to the act of coming out, but they are very different events. Particularly in research and teaching contexts, disclosure is not a freeing act. It becomes a pedagogical necessity so that discussion may be grounded in the here and now.

There may be a passing moment of shock, disgust, or pity, but those are all human visceral responses and should not be judged. Once the moment passes, then and only then may engagement and discussion grounded in the present transform the idea of HIV into something real that impacts individuals. It is something that millions of us who are HIV-positive deal with every day. There is a responsibility in the livability of HIV to acknowledge that not everyone has been as fortunate. Recognizing its importance places today's HIV/AIDS reality on a continuum, positioned somewhere in the middle of the story of AIDS. In turn, declaring the importance of the disease for individuals and on the global stage is the necessary reminder that there is still much work to do: global access to treatment, destigmatization, vaccine, cure. Disclosing one's status is both an opportunity and a responsibility to be a part of the legacy of the AIDS movement, a movement that fought for lives and dignity.

Teaching the American AIDS plays to theatre students is, like disclosure itself, an act that has the potential to help destigmatize an HIV-positive status. Plays are meant to represent real lives. AIDS plays represent lives dealing with illness, pain, marginalization, and survival. A discussion of the plays involves discussing the disease. And discussion, once it begins and grows, is like disclosure. These are acts that cannot ever be undone. Dramaturgical investigation of AIDS in a play means discovering how the AIDS reality of the script differs from the students' world. Students today must reconcile HIV, the manageable chronic condition, preventable but incurable, with depictions of a mysterious fatal illness that insidiously made its way into marginalized communities. This all begins with an excavation of the contemporary understanding of HIV/AIDS. What is known? What is presumed? Where are the gaps in knowledge? What are the contemporary circumstances that might have prevented Michael Friedman from seeking treatment? Then, how is this all different from the world represented in the play? Theatre presents a distinct way of knowing HIV/AIDS in that the relationship between the audience and the text must be newly forged with each encounter – it must be re-forged, or theatre becomes an inert form of art. Theatre is active. It is this re-invention that re-invigorates the individual plays and allows them to deepen the understanding of AIDS for new audiences. Theatre artists encountering AIDS plays for the first time are the ones to breathe new life into those plays. In this, perhaps I am the relic; my students will determine the real use-value of the corpus of AIDS drama.

The AIDS plays are acts of disclosure. Sometimes this act is literal, as in the case of Larry Kramer's sequel to *The Normal Heart*. But often the playwright's disclosure isn't of their own serostatus, but rather it is an implicit declaration that HIV/AIDS is an issue worthy of writing a play about. In the myriad stories that are found in the American AIDS plays, there is a common element that lives are affected by the pandemic. Early plays may not have a name for the disease. Later plays may grapple with memory and continued stigmatization. But regardless of when a play was written, students today must first acknowledge the playwright's individual need to write his, her, or their AIDS play. And eventually, after assessing their own individual and cultural understanding of HIV/AIDS, students must account for the distance between the world of the play and their own. Just as my act of disclosure creates a co-communicative responsibility to explore why HIV status needs a special conversation, studying an AIDS play requires a discussion of the importance of the play's topic – both when it was written and now.

Nothing is better for teaching the act of developing critical consciousness and human generosity than theatre. Because everything that is on stage isn't. And everything that isn't also is. To be drawn into the action of a play is to be a part of it. Having lived through the moment of pure theatrical relationship means accepting the possibility of having been changed as a result. In its momentary life, the play exposes a perfection of transience. This happens to be the thing that I find most exciting as an actor, as an audience member, and as a theatre scholar. The play, on some level, is never finished. It is incomplete and then it's gone forever. Tony Kushner wrote of this ineffable temporality by saying, "We live in a world where we have such a strong relationship to inorganic commodities that pretend to this kind of completion" (Signature Theatre Company). But a play exists for an unrepeatable moment and then endures forever within changeable memory. Perhaps I am a lucky one. I was diagnosed with HIV at a time and in a place of privilege. I was told on the day of my diagnosis that if I take care of myself, I may anticipate a normal life expectancy. "Normal" is a bland word that suddenly meant the world. I lived through times and have passed through places where those facing a similar diagnosis would not have heard the word "normal." In contemplating the ways in which I, as a teacher, might share with my students the ways the AIDS plays teach about the pandemic, I have a responsibility to share my experience – both in living with HIV and in finding my place in the continuum through the AIDS plays. I view this as the performance that follows the performance. The perpetuity of theatre casts ourselves in its continuation. Paul Woodruff describes this type of audience inversion where the watchers become the watched:

> Theater is the art of finding human action worth watching, and it mostly does this by finding human characters worth caring about. We need to practice that art, on both sides – to find people worth watching and, for ourselves, to make ourselves worth watching when we need to be watched ... Willing or not, at one time or another, each of us will be among the watchers and the watched. (22)

If my experience in learning about my acquired history through the theatre is valuable, then it is worth sharing. When that happens in a learning environment, then the experience shifts into action: discussion, conversation, discerning the value of the world of the play. I benefit from the sharing. Martin Buber understands this delightful reality of teaching:

> Relation is reciprocity. My You acts on me as I act on it. Our students teach us, our works inform us. The "wicked" becomes a revelation when they are touched by the sacred basic word. How we are educated by children, by animals! Inscrutably involved, we live in the currents of universal reciprocity. (67)

The theatre is a perfect medium for instruction, as many successful teachers know. To borrow from Stanislavsky, it invites the student to find their magic "if" – if I lived in that moment, if then was now, if there was here. HIV/AIDS is one of the most horrific things to ever happen to this world and its people. As the plays teach of the human impact of the plague, theatre, in its incompleteness, demands a recognition that the age of AIDS is not over.

Students are likely to know AIDS within the frame of sexual health education strategies, and they are likely to have an opinion on HIV stigma, but the phases and events that led to their understanding might not be entirely known. What the corpus of AIDS drama offers that a history textbook cannot is the personal experience of the characters brought to life through the individual relationship built between the student and the play.

The mystique of theatre is often in its ephemerality, that it disappears the moment the curtain falls. But what disappears? It is the living presence of the characters that ceases to exist when the performance ends. AIDS plays are particularly potent in that the vanishing of the life on stage parallels the disappearance of people who died of AIDS. The plays, therefore, are a type of conjuring that calls forth the presence of those who have been lost – a living memorial to the souls claimed by the plague. When the performance ends, it is a sort of reenactment of the loss of those people and a revisiting of the mourning experienced by those left behind. With the AIDS plays, the theatre is simultaneously a place of embodied memorialization and a location of memory.

In her exploration of performance as a utopian enactment, Jill Dolan asks, "Is it too much to ask of performance, that it teach us to love and to link us with the world, as well as to see and to think critically about social relations?" (23). She asks the question to grapple with two distinct modes of theatrical understanding. A play is either viewed as something that draws you in, encouraging an empathetic connection with the characters and action, a source of individual joy and sorrow reflecting one's own state of being in the world, or a play is an object of critical analysis designed to make you think. An AIDS play answers Dolan by saying, "No. It is not too much to ask." One play can make us both feel and think and still send us out into the world ready to effect change. The difficulty in this duality, however, is that it may not do all of that for all people. The experience of sharing time and space with a group of people in an audience does not mean that the individual's experience is duplicated within every member of the audience. Exactly the opposite – we all relate to a play in our own ways. When viewed as the performance of living memorial, the AIDS play answers the complexity of collected mourning by exposing it as an assortment of individual experiences. As the end of the play signals the end of the living memorial and forces the audience to return to their lives, the varied ways in which the individual members of the audience will re-enter the world prevent the play as a memorial from perpetuating a collected melancholia.

While serving to memorialize those who were lost to AIDS and to recall a time that passed, the performance of AIDS plays uniquely handles the outcome of memory and grief. First in scripting the story, the play articulates the loss. Second, in embodying the characters that represent the time, the plays serve as a living connection with that time. Third, through the ephemerality of performance, the conclusion of the play resists an unending cycle of melancholia. Finally, the makeup of audiences at public performances of AIDS plays blurs the demarcation between those who have grieved and those who are too young to have grieved for a time before AIDS. When the members of the audience leave the auditorium, they will individually process their experience with the play. But for the duration of the play, the experience of bearing witness to a time past is shared by all members of the audience. Those for whom the play represents a moment in their lives, one perhaps they have yet to pull through, are seated with people learning about the represented AIDS reality by way of the play.

In this blending, the theatre brings together individuals who need the play for different reasons. The living memorial of the play serves to erase the temporal divisions that separate different audiences affected by HIV/AIDS in different ways.

Finally, and possibly most significantly, regardless of the national setting of the world of the text, plays about AIDS serve an important function in fighting statistical fatigue. It is common, without visible signs of HIV in the daily lives of most Americans (a status quo that often invites those with HIV to conceal their status), the American plays about AIDS serve to personalize the disease. Characters in the plays, both American and otherwise, live with HIV and die from AIDS. This is a consistent embodied reminder that HIV can be anywhere. When considered in conjunction with misconceptions that AIDS is a thing of the past, or a thing that devastates only the developing world, the living presence on stage serves as a potent reminder of the living and current presence of HIV/AIDS throughout the world.

In June 1987, Elizabeth Taylor, the national chairperson of the American Foundation for AIDS Research, made an appearance at a star-studded cocktail party at Sotheby's in New York City to collect a \$400 000 check from art dealer Leo Castelli. The contribution, in Castelli's words, was "just a modest beginning," and the event served as a kick-off for Art Against AIDS (Crimp 5). As Taylor accepted the check, she graciously acknowledged the potential for the art world to contribute more than just money to the fight against AIDS. "Art lives forever" was her idealistic sentiment (Crimp 5). Ostensibly this was a celebration of the possibility that making works of art might raise awareness and create impressions of the plague that would withstand the test of time. There is a perceived durability in some arts, that once the works are complete, they are eternal. But not all art has the same relationship with time. Visual art may endure, but performance is ephemeral. I choose to believe that Taylor wasn't just speaking about visual art. Her platitude inferred that all art needed to live because people were dying. Life in the face of death. Hope instead of despair. The theatre is a place where art is given life. A single play is made anew with every performance. A new production of a familiar play reinvents that play in the here and now. Studying plays should not be merely a practice in recognizing the world of the text. When performed or studied, the American AIDS plays are windows through which the pandemic as it was then and as it is today are mutually illuminated.

Susan Sontag was cynical when she stated her view of what happens when those who believe themselves to be safe regard the pain of others:

> People are often unable to take in the sufferings of those close to them. For all the voyeuristic lure – and the possible satisfaction of knowing – this is not happening to me, I'm not ill, I'm not dying, I'm not trapped in a war – it seems normal for people to fend off thinking about the ordeals of others, even others with whom it would be easy to identify. (*Regarding the Pain of Others*, 99)

On one hand, perhaps in the darkened auditorium, an audience is drawn into voyeurism while watching a play. From a seat in the balcony, an individual audience member may underline their belief that they are safe from HIV infection, that AIDS has no place in their world, and that the time that screamed for activism is ended. This is passivity. Martin Buber might label this as "experience" – unaffected, the individual retains an I-It relationship with the play. But theatre is live; as such, it does not lend itself to passivity. Pedagogically necessary, and perhaps taught through example, the student must not remain passive when encountering an AIDS play. Being truly present means allowing oneself to be affected. Finding one's own place in a play is not just the purview of an actor. All individuals who make the play their own discover the heartbeat of theatrical relationships. Studying theatre means simultaneously observing the life of a play and instilling that play with life: this is an I-You relationship in which both are capable of changing the other. While the takeaway from any play is an individual's enterprise, as a teacher I look to my students and expect their willingness to find themselves in the play. HIV/AIDS is an inescapable part of their world.

Typical undergraduate students are either in, or are about to be in, the age demographic deemed most at risk for HIV infection. I do not profess that a study of the corpus of American AIDS drama is a strategy for prevention. To some individuals, it may serve that function. Since the first appearance of ACT UP's now famous slogan Silence = Death, awareness has always been deemed the first step in fighting HIV/AIDS. Reading the AIDS plays means cultivating an awareness. This cannot be without value. But in its most useful form, studying theater means a meeting of one's own life with the lives depicted in the play. HIV/AIDS becomes a present reality. Retaining its presence then means recalling the lived experience of the play. Like visual art, performance endures in its reinvention. Studying the corpus of drama written about and in response to HIV/AIDS means an enduring consciousness of AIDS.

WORKS CITED

Buber, Martin. *I and Thou*. Translated by Walter Kaufmann. Simon & Schuster, 1970.

Crimp, Douglas, editor. *AIDS Cultural Analysis/Cultural Activism*. MIT Press, 1991.

Dolan, Jill. *Utopia in Performance: Finding Hope in the Theater*. U of Michigan P, 2005.

Kramer, Larry, screenplay. *The Normal Heart*. HBO Films, 2014.

Paulson, Michael. "'Brilliant,' and Lost to AIDS: The Theater World Asks Why." *The New York Times*, 15 Oct. 2017.

Signature Theatre Company. "The Ascent of Angels in America: Signature Theatre Company Celebrates Tony Kushner's Gay Fantasia on National Themes." 2010.

Sontag, Susan. *Illness as Metaphor and AIDS and Its Metaphors*. Ferrar, Straus and Giroux, 1990.

–. *Regarding the Pain of Others*. Picador, 2003.

Woodruff, Paul. *The Necessity of Theater: The Art of Watching and Being Watched*. Oxford UP, 2008.

# PART III

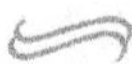

# Exploring Practice-Based Embodied Health Narratives

# 7 Decolonial Feminist Acts of Health/Care in Senegalese Urban Arts

JULIE C. VAN DAM

## Introduction

When *Ecrire l'Afrique-Monde* was published in 2017, it announced itself as a potent remedy against a host of colonial ills. Solidly moored in extra-metropolitan, global southern spaces and clearly committed to writing and writers well beyond the canon, one of the goals of this decolonial project, as editors Achille Mbembe and Felwine Sarr write, is no less than to compel us to "make life habitable," indeed *livable*, "for all" (3). Throughout the collection, decolonial thought is explicitly named as that which catalyzes habitability, healing, and ultimately, *health* itself. But it is in the streets of Dakar, Senegal, Sarr's home country, where one can identify a material and highly visible praxis demanding our attention, one I term "decolonial health/care." In this piece, I argue that contemporary Senegalese urban arts articulate and enact a radical and feminist decolonization of health/care in the public, or common, space. Explored here are the exceedingly present and accessible collaborative arts practices of health activism, or decolonial health/care, seen most notably in the graffiti and hip hop emerging from and located in the neglected outskirts of Dakar such as Pikine and Keur Massar – especially by female actors and their allies.

Since their inception in the late 1980s and even more so today, cultural practices such as graffiti and hip hop in Senegal have defined themselves by their very public presence and their active reclaiming of health outside neocolonial and Western models. This prolific body of work speaks to the exceedingly present and vital collaborative arts practices of health activism, or what I define here as health/care. To be sure, there is a deep history of Senegalese cultural practice that simultaneously names, critiques, *and* reforms bio-social precarity in urban spaces, but female actors and their allies in Senegal have introduced decolonial feminist conversations, activism, and cultural practices around health, bodily integrity, and security. Using as a case study two female graffiti artists and the collective Gënji Hip Hop, it becomes clear that these works exemplify "theory from the south" in the way that Jean and John Comaroff mean. These artists effectively rewrite the script that limits the Global South – but especially women – to passive victims of the processes of neo-liberalization (Fredericks; Mbembe and Nuttall). If, for Achille Mbembe, decolonization is defined "as a praxis of self-defense and as an experience of emergence and uprising" (*Out of the Dark Night* 224), I would argue that women in the Global South are even more potent actors of decolonization given their relationships to an intersecting set of categories that "hierarchically organise notions of human worth" (Kolářová and Wiedlack 126) such as but not limited to race, gender, class, health, ability, sexuality, political and cultural affiliations, and even economic productivity.

**Bio-social Precarity within the Common**

The intertwined legacies of patriarchal colonization, neocolonialism and neo-liberalism in Senegal have catalyzed a spectrum of health/care urban arts proffered more and more frequently from female actors and their allies. In adopting the notion of health/care, I wish to align these artist-activists with a broader view of what constitutes not only health concerns (what is worthy of attention or even diagnosis) but also (health)care outside a Western biomedical framework. Referencing the work of Jane Gross, Adriana Petryna, and Joao Biehlon on what might be broadly termed biomedical citizenship, Jean Comaroff rightly asks, "Why is it that, in many places, access to medicine – rather than, say, jobs, clean air, or freedom from war – has come to epitomize citizenship, equity, and justice?" (206). To be sure, much of the work emerging from these women artist-activists implicitly poses the same question. But before turning my gaze there, I will trace the connections between, on the one hand, understandings of health, disease, and debility in the Global South and, on the other, feminist praxis within said spaces. While this chapter does not mean to address disability and cripness within Senegalese urban arts, it would be irresponsible to read health and bio-precarity outside disability.

In their recent edited collection on disability in Africa, Toyin Falola and Nic Hamel invoke Julie Livingston's early intervention on debility in the African context to conclude that "global structures of neocolonialism, racism, economic injustice, and ecological catastrophe produce and maintain disability throughout the Global South through processes of debilitation that often go unnoticed" (30). Although the explicit focus of Falola and Hamel's intervention is "disability in Africa," this observation is patently true of a multitude of bodily and mental states that include not just disability but debility, vulnerability, and precarity. If Judith Butler does not mention health, illness, or disability explicitly in her early work on vulnerability and precarity, her later dialogue with Jasbir Puar proves useful here. In the context of neo-liberalism's extractive demands, Butler says that "precarity is indissociable from that dimension of politics that addresses the organization and protection of bodily needs" (170). While feminist disability philosopher Margrit Shildrick reads this as bio-precarity, I would apply to the Senegalese context Kateřina Kolářova's broader term of bio-social precarity. These are not necessarily spectacular or official or even diagnosable health or bodily states. As Stephen Knadler has shown in the context of the twentieth-century United States, "everyday, slow, debilitating, contagious, and toxic attrition" of Black health went for the most part ignored in the face of the more explicit risks posed by White supremacist thinking (3). Replace this "explicit risk" with malaria, yellow fever, and/or COVID-19, and it applies to a slew of African nations in the Global South. Knadler's foci are the "gradual, toxic, and everyday assaults" of racial violence "that occurred through unsanitary housing, polluted drinking water, unequal segregated healthcare, the absence of sewage lines, unsafe food, or traumatic environmental stress" (4) that echo many of the daily realities in Senegal. But added to that are also the threats of gender-based traumas.

Recent theoretical interventions on decolonial feminism do not address health or precarity in any sustained way, but they do gesture towards it. For Françoise Vergès, decolonial feminism productively counters what she has recently coined "civilizational feminism," one which inherently supports and exacerbates "the perpetuation of domination based on class, gender and race" (3–4) and, I would add, normative ideas of health and ability. To open Vergès's 2019 *A Decolonial Feminism* is to see how the spectre of health and precarity haunts the decolonial feminist project without being given full entry. In her brief introduction, Vergès tells a story meant to frame her project: that of the 2018 strike by "racialized and overexploited" female union members who clean the Gare du Nord train station in Paris (2). Vergès rightly insists on the very unhealthful nature of this work, which creates "these precarious lives, these endangered lives, these worn-out bodies" (2). The irony of their labour (maintaining hygienic conditions for travellers while being subjected to regular debilitation via physical depletion and noxious cleaning products) goes unremarked by Vergès, but it merits attention. To be sure, in Dakar, the historical legacy of what I have termed elsewhere *hygiaesthetics*, has played an undeniable role in the proliferation of public urban arts addressing health and/or the body.

Tracing the decolonial and health/care praxis of these works means attending to the deeply embedded colonial histories that haunt Senegal and especially Senegalese women (Mbembe, "Time and Event" 2003). If Mbembe was speaking here to the "deeply embedded" traumas expressed by writers such as Ken Bugul, his metaphor extends to the multiple ways in which minds and bodies bear the imprints of a long history and tangible present of rhetorical and material precarization through colonization and globalization. One of the key reasons that the cityscapes of Dakar and its outskirts have come to be punctuated by these material interventions, whether visual, sonic, and/or tactile, has to do with its complex and sometimes conflictual histories *as* a post/colonial urban space. Emerging from colonial rule, it seemed and still seems, Senegal has seen at once a series of erasures and excessive fabrications in attempting to establish its place among "healthy" and "able" African nations. By using these terms, I mean precisely to evoke the Western models that continue to determine the desirability, viability, respectability and *investability* of the Global South.

In Senegal, the two-centuries-long violence of colonization by the French, lasting from the seventeenth century to 1960, set the stage for the regime of Léopold Sédar Senghor. Under Senghor, the 1960s and 1970s witnessed the neo-colonial, state-sponsored forced disappearance of a host of ill and/or disabled citizens from the city streets seen as "human obstructions," "undesirables," and "human garbage [*déchets humains*]" in the guise of fabricating purportedly healthful and appealing or "hygiaesthetic" public spaces for French tourists and dignitaries (Nack Ngue 103-6; Van Dam). While many of those who were rounded up and placed outside the city limits in colonial-era labour camps had visible or explicit impairments or health conditions (whether physical, mental, or cognitive), many others (who are also of deep concern to urban artists) dwelled and dwell today still in varying degrees of health insecurity. To be sure, the post-independence policies of erasure were compounded by structural adjustment policies of the 1980s and 90s which reduced debt but demanded major cuts to social services such as healthcare. And, finally, with the emergence of neoliberal global capitalism, what has resulted is a deeply entrenched bio-social precarity.

And one of the contributors to the slow but steady debilitation of its citizens is precisely (still) its gleaming hyperbolic cityscape. Since the early 2000s, Dakar has seen "une boulimie urbanistique ("an urbanistic bulimia") (Diouf and Fredericks 19, my translation): mammoth, overly visible, and concrete (or sometimes metallic) signs of economic and national health in the shape of national monuments, a series of slick toll routes, a glitzy new airport, a new soccer stadium, and even a futuristic city, Diamniadio Lake City forty kilometres south of Dakar. These "grands projets" have been executed with astonishing speed and, as Abdourahmane Seck notes, regardless of the price tag, the necessary diversion of public funds, the environmental damage, or the human cost. Rosalind Fredericks explains that "radically uneven, sporadic, and performative investments in urban infrastructure left parts of the city to rot, rust, and slowly crumble with the passage of time while others were spiffed up with elite, world-class urban aesthetics" (10). Much work has yet to be done on the very real environmental and human costs of this intense and uneven urban development. What I aim to do here is not to enumerate these costs but to expose the critiques of them that, in their own ways, lay claim to the public space. Dakar is indeed a city layered in scaffolding. In acknowledging this, Felwine Sarr writes that "within all the various construction sites of our cities, we must leave room for creative spaces: unfinished sites that represent the possibles" (109). If we seek out and lend attention to the urban arts of health/care, however, we can identify a host of "possibles" in and among the common spaces of the city.

If for Lauren Berlant, precarity, or as I argue bio-social precarity, "is a rallying cry for a thriving new world of interdependency and care that's *not just private*" (Puar 166, my emphasis) then in Senegal the creation of this "new world" is not just present but active, redundant, and even chronic. As Butler says, "When the bodies of those deemed 'disposable' assemble in public view, they are saying, 'We have not slipped quietly into the shadows of public life; we have not become *the glaring absence* that structures your public life'" (Puar 168, my emphasis). Against this glaring absence, these female actors perform quotidien acts of bodily, artistic, and activist *presence* within the common (public) space.

It is not incidental that Senegalese anthropologist and historian Abdourahmane Seck employs health metaphors to diagnose the political malfeasance that has characterized Senegalese politics since the election of Abdoulaye Wade in 2000, through the presidency of Macky Sall (2012–24). Referenced earlier, Seck's critique is focused in part on the misallocation of funds to produce a dazzling cityscape at the expense of its citizens and the environment. What has resulted, Seck suggests, are deep fractures in the common space and the community, both material and metaphorical. The title of Seck's piece alone merits some dissection: the original French "Panser l'en-commun" could be translated metaphorically as "Healing the in-common" or, more literally and more *materially*, as "Bandaging the in-common." The healing-bandaging that Seck invokes is one that quite literally sutures the gaps between seemingly disparate bodies and subjectivities. Seck explains that his work seeks to unearth "des zones de touche pour sutures, de réparation de soi et de l'Autre" ("zones of contact for *sutures* that repair the individual and the Other") (311–12, my emphasis and translation). To arrive here at these "zones of contact" within the "in-common," Seck turns to the Senegalese (Wolof) notion of *mbokk*. He explains: "Au Sénégal, le mot *mbokk* dit à la fois parenté et partage, mais aussi *inclusion* ("In Senegal, the word *mbokk* signifies at once family and sharing, but also *inclusion*" (332, my emphasis and translation). Aligned with ideas of community, contact, exchange, and capaciousness, this cultural principle is one that imbues the quotidien and, what is more, informs and catalyzes it. Achille Mbembe goes further here. Drawing on Frantz Fanon, he links the space of the hospital – the patient prostrate, the sterility, the surrender to medical intervention, the division between medical caregiver and patient – as one that can hinder such "communing" and communication. And yet that it is precisely in the "constitution of a common realm" that actual care and healing can emerge (*Necropolitics* 153). To be sure, the practice of reclaiming the streets *is* an act of constitution, or as Mamadou Bâ contends, it represents "la réécriture du récit de l'en-commun" ("the rewriting of the narrative of the in-common") (para. 1, my translation).

Up and against the Western desire for edifices of verticality, separation, and closed-off-ness, Felwine Sarr contends that inhabitants of African cities such as Dakar "choose to privilege these other interstices where we can encounter each other, where we live and where we do so fully" (110). Moving beyond Seck's application, a deeper study of the root word *bokk* – to participate (Faye) – reveals that praxis is absolutely fundamental to *mbokk*. What becomes clear in the work of female urban artists in Dakar is precisely this sense of redundant and persistent production of materiality and meaning that is always already dialogic. It is as much a repetitive practice of politically engaged art-making as it is an exchange with the viewer or participant.

### From Set Setal to Feminist Arts

The urban artistic practice of graffiti and murals has played a crucial role in establishing Dakar as an ongoing site for accessible, public interventions into health and health/care. To be sure, the preponderance of female cultural actors today who are producing works against health precarity represent a much more active, visible, and prolific iteration of the

Set Setal movement that emerged in the late 1980s when Dakarois youth, frustrated with the state and its literal *and* political filth, initiated Set Setal (meaning "To be clean, To clean up" in Wolof). With Dakar being termed by one newspaper as "la capitale de la saleté" ("the capital of filth)" and "de plus en plus insécure ("more and more unsafe") (Bugnicourt and Diallo 49), Set Setal represented a kind of urban restoration and renewal that combined the removal of waste and other health hazards (including barriers to access) with the addition of murals and graffiti, the vast majority of which – 17 percent across 14 different themes – addressed "saleté-santé" ("filth-health") (Bugnicourt and Diallo 27).

According to historian Mamadou Diouf's words, in Set Setal, "the iconography is reformulated, giving a new dimension to a message (on hygiene, vaccinations, treating and preventing diarrhea) that the project *Santé pour Tous en l'An 2000* [Health for All in the Year 2000] had outlined but failed to popularize" ("(Re)Imagining an African City" 359). Neither this exhaustive plan, launched in 1979 by the World Health Organization (Regional Committee for the Western Pacific), nor the Bamako Initiative, launched in 1987 in the wake of structural readjustment, made any real tangible impact in Senegal where many of the proposed interventions were never fully implemented. Mamadou Bâ rightly underscores the sociopolitical impact of these movements, for these prolific graffiti-murals inaugurated a very public intervention into health, well-being, and security for average citizens moving through the cityscape whether by bus, by foot, or by assistive mobility device. But ultimately, Set Setal was subjected to a neocolonial impulse of discipline; it was co-opted by Dakar's then mayor in an effort to contain the activists and channel their energies (and active bodies) into productive labour (Fredericks 9).

If, as Diouf contends, the Set Setal movement enacted "a radical transformation of the idea of citizenship" in part through the "conflation of domestic and public spheres" ("Engaging Postcolonial Cultures" 3) and for Bâ, it allowed for a "appropriation spatiale et générationnelle du lien social" ("spatial and generational appropriation of social ties") (para. 10, my translation), then for today's urban female artists, the "spatial appropriation" of Dakar has become deeply imbued with a radical political positionality. As our case studies make clear, it is in the regular contact between artist and art, on the one hand, and art and participants, on the other, that the common can emerge. As prolific graffiti artist Docta explains, graffiti allows one to "rentrer dans le quotidien de n'importe qui" ("enter into the daily life of no matter whom") (2018). While much of the graffiti today is still produced by male artists, a growing number of women are making themselves and their personal concerns for health/care – bodily and health security for themselves and others – present in the public space.

Vergès rightly locates the origins of decolonial feminisms in the Global South. Even more pointed, Sylvia Tamale's *Decolonization and Afro-Feminism* means to "construct a counter-hegemonic feminist narrative" (21). Both Tamale and Vergès want to revise the decades-long processes of effacement and disavowal in discussions about feminism in the Global South, and by so doing respond to Ella Shohat's 2001 claim that "these antipatriarchal and even, at times, antiheterosexist subversions within anticolonial struggles remain marginal to the global feminist canon" (1269–70). As Wasso Tounkara, co-founder of the Dakar-based feminist urban arts collective Gënji Hip Hop expressed in a recent interview, feminism is deeply intertwined with an exceptionally broad view of health and rights; she defines it as "le bien-être et l'autonomie des femmes" ("the well-being and autonomy of women" (Wasso). While Knadler does not focus exclusively on Black women, his consideration of the broader context of crip, anti-racist activism in the United States is useful for reading decolonial health/care praxis well beyond American borders. For example, he looks at Black leaders and community activists who "were trying less to cure, fix, or remake the disabled and distressed as normal assimilated citizens than to create new ecologies for giving people what they needed and to cultivate *well-being*" (4, my emphasis). For women like Wasso Tounkara and hip hop artist Mina la voilée, health can and should encompass physical, mental, and environmental well-being as well as personal autonomy. As Tounkara noted, "Quand je dis 'Je suis en santé,' je veux dire que j'ai la liberté de penser, d'agir" ("When I say, 'I am healthy,' I mean that I am free to think, to act") (Wasso). Although I explore Mina la voilée's work more in depth elsewhere, she is one of the most prolific voices in feminist hip hop activism today, decolonizing health/care by critiquing heteropatriarchal colonial legacies impacting everything from abusive practices of female incarceration to skin whitening to domestic sexual abuse. Mina explained two separate women's health interventions that were still on the docket, having been delayed by the pandemic. In one, she and other female artists will visit the notoriously deplorable women's prison at Liberté 6 – armed with health and hygiene products – to host a series of workshops on rap and graffiti. While this intervention has yet to take place, there is much graffiti already in Dakar that performs similar decolonial interventions.

As a researcher on the ground in Dakar, to ask which female graffiti artists are producing work around issues of health, illness, and/or disability is to be directed first to one of the founding fathers of Senegalese graffiti, Amadou Lamine Ngom, or Docta, for "Doctor of the Walls." Part of the Doxandem Squad of graffiti artists, Docta's work and legacy are foundational to the contemporary interventions by women such as Zeinixx (born Dieynaba Sidibe), called Senegal's "first lady of graffiti" by her male colleagues (Zeinixx) and Thiat Graff and Dasha'Art, part of the newer generation of artists working across the cityscape of Dakar and beyond.

By far the most well-known and most visible female graffiti artist, Zeinixx is a regular participant in the annual month-long Graff et Santé [Graffiti and Health] festival, founded by Docta in 2008 to bring life to "tous les lieux abandonnés" ("all those places that have been abandoned") (Docta). As conceived by Docta, Graff et Santé is a grassroots, extra-governmental intervention to bring messaging and material change to the lives of Dakarois in the marginalized outskirts of the capital like Pikine. When in an interview (Docta) I asked about support from the Senegalese government, Docta spat out in English (a first in our conversation): "Fuck that shit." Then, in French, "Je ne compte pas sur le gouvernement." ("I don't count on the government"). Instead, he and the artists with whom he works – including Zeinixx – count on the collaboration of those who are in need of health/care, the community members. As Docta explained, they reach out to a specific locality, discuss with inhabitants which health concerns are most pressing, bring in *Médecins sans frontières* (Doctors Without Borders) to inform and treat these concerns while the artists attack the walls, as it were, with art meant to inform on and catalyze health promotion and disease prevention for passersby. Docta spoke of an extended collaboration between the community, the graffiti artists, and the healthcare workers. This allows for health/care not only for the graffiti crew as they learn what illnesses, diseases, or health conditions concern each specific community, but also for those same community members as they meet with healthcare workers and acquire the terms useful to interpreting their health in a biomedical context but outside a capitalist framework. The motto of Graff et Santé, "Santé amoul prix," a mashup of French and Wolof (the majority indigenous language spoken in Senegal), translates to "Health has no price." Aligned with a decolonial health/care model, services are offered free of charge (Doxandem Squad). Of course, these services are limited both temporally (within the festival) and geographically (within the locality) and culturally (by the ethos and objectives of Doctors Without Borders).

But the graffiti, for its part, maintains an active presence that is not only for the inhabitants but quite literally for *any* passerby. And pass they do, especially when the murals or art are situated in highly trafficked areas or thoroughfares for those coming from outside of said locality. In the case of female artists, the act of *production* is also a defiant act of presence. Every artist I have spoken with made it clear that to produce graffiti (or hip hop) as a woman is to be hyper aware of one's body within a space and within an artistic practice normally reserved for men. Thiat Graff and Dasha'Art have negotiated nighttime painting or hooded (or otherwise camouflaged) painting. This wilful invisibility has allowed them more bodily and aesthetic flexibility, vitality, and candour. But like Zeinixx, they also paint very visibly as women precisely to show solidarity with other female artists and artists-to-be. While discussing an upcoming project at an all-girls high school, Zeinixx echoes Tounkara's call for personal autonomy: "My refrain is to tell young people: 'Don't let others choose for you what you would like to do tomorrow'" (Crowe). This kind of active dialogic and embodied presence of being *for the other* evokes the radical decolonial ethos inherent in Frantz Fanon's therapeutic processes. As Mbembe writes, such processes included "new experiences of the body, of movement, of being-together – and even of communion, as the shared commonality that is most alive and vulnerable in humanity" (*Necropolitics* 5)

This constant redundant presence is even more apparent in the most recent interventions by women because they have emerged not only outside organized festivals and often in prominent locations in and around Dakar but also well beyond conventional understandings of what constitutes illness and health. As outlined on their Google Arts & Culture site (Doxandem Squad), the objectives of Graff et Santé are for the most part very tightly organized around specific, identifiable, and diagnosable diseases and health conditions (some diseases they address are malaria, yellow fever, and HIV/AIDS to name a few). While this allows for more targeted interventions, it can also inadvertently neglect the quotidien processes of debilitation that produce bio-social precarity especially among women. In recent interviews, women working in graffiti have expressed frustration at the shift of attention away from "everything else" and solely towards COVID-19 (Thiat Graff, Dasha'Art). And there were a multitude of murals as well as more informal graffiti art interventions that dotted the cityscape of Dakar in the wake of the pandemic – that had nothing to do with COVID-19. As Thiat Graff, one of only two women with RBS Crew (a large and prolific graffiti collective), expressed, "La Covid nous aveugle à toutes les autres maladies et à tous les autres problèmes" ("Covid blinds us to all of the other illnesses and all of the other problems," 2021). What Thiat Graff – *Thiat* meaning "little sister" in Wolof – suggests here is far from a mimicry of her older brothers. "All of the other illnesses and all of the other problems," broad and undefined and quotidian, are precisely what many of these female artists understand intimately and address in their works.

Zeinixx has her studio at Centre Africulturban, a vibrant multi-use space that houses artists studios, classroom space, a training centre, and a performance space in the outsized, neglected department of Pikine outside Dakar. Founded by the well-established hip hop artist Matador in 2006 after a series of particularly devastating floods, he meant it from the beginning to be a space of activism, renewal, and healing through collective artistic interventions. The health impact of these regular floods – regular precisely because of the hasty and ill-conceived construction of Pikine by French colonial authorities in 1952 – is well documented and has been the subject of other artists, including crip/care-focused filmmaker Moly Kane whose first Senegal-based short from 2015 "Guinaw Rails au bout" ("Guinaw Rails at its limit," Guinaw Rails being Kane's own neighbourhood in Pikine) documented – without dialogue – the dangerous, laborious, and seemingly futile removal of dank floodwater from local dwellings, mainly by women. Born and raised in the neighbourhood of Thioraye in Pikine, Zeinixx has experienced first-hand the bio-social precarity inherent there, and her work is clearly aligned with health/care. She has a wide range of health-focused graffiti projects under her belt, from more recognizable health concerns to broader, less specific, and less visible ones. Her largest work in Dakar is notable because it quite literally surrounds the Centre Africulturban, gracing the fifteen-metre (fifty-foot) wall at its entrance, it reads STOP SIDA (STOP AIDS) in her characteristic graff font and bright pastel colour palette. Like all of her graffs, the words are also spelled out in a traditional text font above it. If not all can read either font, its imagery reveals its intent. It should be noted that the extremely low rate of HIV/AIDS cases in Senegal is an anomaly in West Africa, attributed by researchers in part to the numerous public art interventions promoting condom use and testing. One of her other pieces, GEUN, meaning "Better to prevent than to treat" (my translation), aligns with her general approach to health promotion that is holistic and that defies conventional models of clinical care.

## Conclusion

If, for Docta, graffiti is "le trait d'union" [the hyphen] between the people and (their) health, Zeinixx herself seems to be another kind of hyphen. In a recent interview, she explained that her mother had told her to become a doctor. While her chosen profession seems far from the practice of medicine, Zeinixx sees it otherwise, explaining that she basically exchanged "la seringue du médecin pour les outils de la graffeuse" [the syringe of the doctor for the tools of the *graffeuse*, the female graffiti artist] (Zeinixx). She insisted on this point, saying "C'est le graff qui soigne" ("It's graffiti that heals") – herself and others. What Zeinixx suggests here aligns well with a broader cultural approach to health that always already contains within it a notion of the common. As explained by Wolof poet Tijan M. Sallah, health is conceived of relationally, and begins with the definition of "human," or *nit* in Wolof:

> *nit* is a living bundle containing *hel* (mind/intelligence), *yaram* (body), *fit* (courage) and *sagoe* (will; that which balances the self). If any of these elements is absent or goes out of balance, a person is sick. Sickness is, therefore, a social and psychological imbalance, not only a physical one. (24)

Sallah further explains that the "*nit* operates in a social universe [with] great emphasis on social belonging" (24). The common saying *nit nitai garabam* is even more illustrative of this and parallels the words of Zeinixx: "a person is the medicine of another person" (24).

Indeed, both Zeinixx and Wasso Tounkara of Gënji Hip Hop refer to their positionality as one of vigilance followed by action. For Tounkara being a feminist activist means being "dans une position d'alerte" ("in a position of alertness") when there are conditions to "remedy" in society, but particularly for women (Wasso). For Zeinixx's part, when asked about her focus on specific diseases, she replied: "J'observe beaucoup. Je suis alertée par tout" ("I observe a lot. I am alerted by everything") (Zeinixx). The scope of their attention, as these responses suggest, is broad, expansive, and generous; it is not limited to institutionally defined or well-publicized (women's) health conditions. As Sylvia Tamale points out, the connection between feminist activism and physical and mental health is recursive. She writes: "While all activists, regardless of gender, face similar challenges, for women juggling feminist engagement, activism (whether frontline or intellectual) and unpaid family/community care under neoliberal pressures stretches the limits of human capacity and endurance" (248). These artist-activists propulse a decolonial health/care that is deeply invested in the common, or *mbokk*. They are the beating heart of the praxis of what Achille Mbembe theorizes as: the "*active will to community*," which he then explains "is another name for what could be called the *will to life*" (*Out of the Dark Night* 2–3, his emphasis).

## WORKS CITED

*Africulturban*. https://africulturban.wordpress.com/africulturban/. Accessed 6 June 2022.

Bâ, Mamadou. "Dakar, du mouvement Set Setal à Y'en a marre (1989–2012)." *Itinéraires: Littératures, Textes, Cultures*, vol. 1, 2016, pp. 1–12. Special issue: "Ecrire et créer avec les villes en movement."

Bugnicourt, Jacques, and Amadou Diallo. *Set Setal: des murs qui parlent. Nouvelle culture urbaine à Dakar*. ENDA, 1991.

Comaroff, Jean. "Beyond Bare Life: AIDS, (Bio)Politics, and the Neoliberal Order." *The Journal of Popular Culture*, vol. 19, no. 1, 2007, pp. 197–219. https://doi.org/10.1215/08992363-2006-030.

Comaroff, Jean, and John L. *Theory from the South or How Euro-America Is Evolving Toward Africa*. Routledge, 2012.

Crowe, Portia. "Painting a Bigger Picture: Senegal's Pioneering First Lady of Graffiti." *The Guardian*, 10 Jan. 2022, https://www.theguardian.com/global-development/2022/jan/10/painting-a-bigger-picture-senegals-pioneering-first-lady-of-graffiti.

Dasha'Art. Personal interview. 31 Aug. 2021.

Diouf, Mamadou. "Engaging Postcolonial Cultures: African Youth and Public Space." *African Studies Review*, vol. 46, no. 2, 2003, pp. 1–12. https://doi.org/10.2307/1514823.

–. "(Re)Imagining an African City: Performing Culture, Arts, and Citizenship in Dakar (Senegal), 1980–2000." *The Spaces of the Modern City: Imaginaries, Politics, and Everyday Life*, edited by Gyan Prakash and Kevin M. Kruse, Princeton UP, 2008, pp. 346–72.

Diouf, Mamadou, and Rosalind Fredericks, editors. *Les Arts de la citoyenneté: Espaces contestés et civilités urbaines*. Karthala, 2013.

Docta. Personal interview. 2 Jul. 2018.

Doxandem Squad. "Graff et Santé: Santé amoul prix." *Google Arts & Culture Exhibit Page*. https://artsandculture.google.com/exhibit/graff-et-sant%C3%A9/wQsqS6EC. Accessed 27 Sep. 2021.

Falola, Toyin, and Nic Hamel, editors. *Disability in Africa: Inclusion, Care, and the Ethics of Humanity*. Boydell & Brewer, 2021, https://doi.org/10.2307/j.ctv136bz27.

Faye, Saliou. *Micro-dico: Français-Wolof*. IFAN, 1996.

Fredericks, Rosalind. *Garbage Citizenship: Vital Infrastructures of Labor in Dakar, Senegal*. Duke UP, 2018.

Graff, Thiat. Personal interview. 30 Aug. 2021.

Kane, Moly, director. *Guinaw Rails au bout*. Babubu Productions, 2015.

Knadler, Stephen. *Vitality Politics: Health, Debility and the Limits of Black Emancipation*. U of Michigan P, 2019.

Kolářová, Katerina. "'Grandpa Lives in Paradise Now': Biological Precarity and the Global Economy of Debility." *The Feminist Review*, vol. 111, 2015, pp. 75–87. https://doi.org/10.1057/fr.2015.45.

Kolářová, Katerina, and M. Katharina Wiedlack. "Introduction: Crip Notes on the Idea of Development." *Somatechnics: Journal of Bodies – Technologies – Power*, vol. 6, no. 2, 2016, pp. 125–41. Special issue: "Cripping Development." https://www.researchgate.net/publication/345804998_Crip_Notes_on_the_Idea_of_Development/fulltext/6009ced792851c13fe2a7f59/Crip-Notes-on-the-Idea-of-Development.pdf.

Mbembe, Achille. "Time and Event in New Francophone African Narratives." 16 Apr. 2003, UCLA.

–. *Necropolitics.* Translated by Steve Corcoran, Duke UP, 2019.

–. *Out of the Dark Night: Essays on Decolonization.* Translated by Daniela Ginsburg, Columbia UP, 2021.

Mbembe, Achille, and Nuttall, Sarah. "Writing the World from an African Metropolis." *Public Culture*, vol. 16, no. 3, 2004, pp. 347–72. https://doi.org/10.1215/08992363-16-3-347.

Mbembe, Achille, and Felwine Sarr, editors. *Ecrire l'Afrique-Monde*. Philippe Rey / Jimsaan, 2017.

Nack Ngue, Julie. "Toward a New Aesthetic of the Global: Grotesque Bodies, Circulation and Haunting in Fama Diagne Sene's *Le Chant des tênènbres* and Ken Bugul's *La Folie et la mort*." *Critical Conditions: Disability and Illness in Francophone African and Caribbean Women's Writing.* Lexington Books, 2012.

Puar, Jasbir. "Precarity Talk: A Virtual Roundtable with Lauren Berlant, Judith Butler, Bojana Cvejic, Isabell Lorey, Jasbir Puar, and Ana Vujanovic." *TDR: The Drama Review*, vol. 56, no. 4, winter 2012; pp. 163–77. https://doi.org/10.1162/DRAM_a_00221.

Regional Committee for the Western Pacific. *Global Strategy for Health for All by the Year 2000.* World Health Organization, 1981. http://iris.wpro.who.int/handle/10665.1/6967.

Sallah, Tijan M. *Wolof: Senegal.* Rosen Publishing Group, 1996.

Sarr, Felwine. *Afrotopia.* Translated by Drew Burke and Sarah Jones-Boardman, U of Minnesota P, 2019.

Seck, Abdourahmane. "Panser l'en-commun: Contribution à une forfaiture politique au Sénégal." *Ecrire l'Afrique-Monde*, edited by Achille Mbembe and Felwine Sarr. Jimsaan, 2017, pp. 307-40.

Shildrick, Margrit. "Neoliberalism and Embodied Precarity: Some Crip Responses." *The South Atlantic Quarterly*, vol. 118, no. 3, pp. 595–613, https://doi.org/10.1215/00382876-7616175.

Shohat, Ella. "Area Studies, Transnationalism, and the Feminist Production of Knowledge." *Signs*, vol. 26, no. 4, 2001, pp. 1269–72.

Tamale, Sylvia. *Decolonization and Afro-Feminism.* Daraja Press, 2020.

Tounkara, Wasso. Personal Interview. 1 Sep. 2021.

Van Dam, Julie. "Re-viewing Disability in Postcolonial West Africa: Ousmane Sembène's Early Resistant Bodies in *Xala*." *The Journal of Literary and*

*Cultural Disability Studies*, vol. 10, no. 2, 2016, pp. 207–21, https://doi.org/10.3828/jlcds.2016.17.
Vergès, Françoise. *A Decolonial Feminism*. Translated by Ashley J. Bohrer with the author, Pluto Press, 2021.
Zeinixx. Personal interview. 3 Sep. 2021.

# 8 "We Are Not Waiting": When Patients Become Medical Innovators

AUDE BANDINI AND JONATHAN GARFINKEL

## The Burden of Diabetes, Evolutions in Technology, and DIYAPS

Up until a century ago, a type 1 diabetes (T1D) diagnosis was a death sentence. In this autoimmune disease, insulin producing cells in the pancreas are irreversibly destroyed. The lives of people living with T1D (PWT1D) were forever changed when insulin was discovered and extracted in the laboratories of the University of Toronto. Since Banting and Best's discovery in 1921, the quality of insulins has improved and become faster acting and RNA derived (as opposed to beef or pork derivatives), and the delivery more efficient and precise. For some, injections have been replaced by insulin pumps, small pager-sized devices that release insulin through tubing into a catheter inserted under the skin. Technologies for measuring blood glucose, too, have changed by leaps and bounds, from a urine-test stick to home blood glucose meters to continuous glucose monitors (CGM), small copper-wired sensors that measure interstitial fluid and send the results to a smartphone every five minutes. In spite of these developments, including greater knowledge and understanding of diet, pancreatic function, and diabetes lifestyle, the burden of managing diabetes still depends on taking insulin, which involves a multitude of decisions and calculation strategies by the patient (Feudtner).

Living with diabetes is a precarious balancing act of managing insulin dosages against blood glucose levels, taking into account myriad factors including carbohydrate intake, exercise and stress. Taking too much insulin can result in hypoglycaemia, which, if left untreated, can lead to coma or death. Taking too little insulin can lead to hyperglycaemia, which causes a variety of long-term complications, including kidney failure, blindness, and heart attack. The complexities of living with diabetes are many, and the dangers numerous, leading to an underexplored area of mental health side effects, including anxiety and depression (Liu et al.).

Relieving the burden of care is a prevalent concern within the diabetes community and emerging within the pharmaceutical and tech worlds (Braune et al., "Real-World Use"). Among other fields of research, including hormone and gene transplant therapy, the goal to take the human calculation out of the equation for insulin therapy is a leading ambition in diabetes research (Cleal et al.). To do this involves creating a system in which the CGM and insulin pump communicate in real time with each other, using a computer algorithm to decide how much or how little insulin the patient requires. This artificial pancreas, or closed-loop system, is considered the "holy grail" of diabetes treatment and research. Yet while the technology for such a system has existed for a decade, closed-loop devices have only just recently come onto the market. This is due to a number of factors, including lengthy clinical trials required by health regulators and patent proprietary ambitions of industry (Garfinkel, "Hacking Diabetes"). Interoperability among competing medical devices is not a model companies are used to working with, and health industry regulators are slow, bureaucratic beasts.

Born out of patient frustration with the medical device industry and government health agencies, do-it-yourself artificial pancreas systems (DIYAPS) have emerged. DIYAPS grew out of the patient-run Nightscout Project, whose focus was on ownership of personal data and the need for parents of children with T1D to access CGM data to monitor nighttime glucose levels before it was possible to do so on market sold devices (Gottlieb and Cluck). In developing several remote technologies, and sharing them online as open source, Nightscout set a standard for open-source activities within the diabetes world, including DIYAPS. Using the hashtag #WeAreNotWaiting, a global online community emerged (Lee et al.).

Practically speaking, DIYAPS began in 2010, when San Francisco programmer and person with diabetes Ben West discovered a security flaw in his Medtronic insulin pump. During his off-hours from work, over the course of several years, he found a way to remotely control his insulin pump through Bluetooth, posting his results online. Around the same time, Dana Lewis and Scott Leibrand experimented and developed computer algorithms that could calculate how much insulin a pump should administrate in response to real-time blood glucose, based on past interpretations of CGM data and future predictions (Lewis is also a PWT1D). Combining this algorithm with West's discovery, they created a "smart" system that could take the complicated gamut of hourly decisions out of the patient's hands, calculating and delivering insulin on the patient's behalf. Using a Raspberry Pi to communicate between devices, Lewis and Leibrand created Open APS; around the same time, Pete Schwamb developed the more user-friendly Loop for the iPhone (his daughter Riley is a PWT1D). By 2015, the DIYAPS movement was well underway. Today, there are three open-source, closed-loop systems: Open APS, Android APS, and Loop (Garfinkel, "Hacking Diabetes").

According to Health Canada guidelines, a medical device needs federal approval if it is to be sold for profit (Garfinkel, "Hacking Diabetes"). To circumvent regulators like Health Canada, the European Medicines Agency, and the US Food and Drug Administration (FDA), DIYAPS require the PWT1D to build their own app, thereby turning thousands of T1D into hackers (Gottlieb and Cluck). The components required to set up the iOS-based Loop cost USD 150 for a mini Bluetooth LE radio (plus postage and handling, assembly not included), an Apple developer's licence (USD 100), an iPhone, a Mac computer (which isn't necessary for all systems now), and the patience to follow the instructions available on Facebook for how to build the app. Computer illiterate people, including the authors of this chapter, are following such instructions – and entrusting their lives to these systems. We both live through and thanks to such innovations in technologies.

Thanks to DIYAPS, a legal grey zone has emerged, challenging current standards of medical care and device regulation. As both authors of this chapter are PWT1D living on DIYAPS, we believe we offer an unusual vantage point, both from experience and through scholarly reflection. We are also aware that this is a movement born of its time. When one of the authors first joined the Looped Facebook group in 2018, there were 2000 members. Now there are over 30 000 members and counting. And while there are currently several "official" closed-loop systems available on the market as of writing this chapter – including the Medtronic 770, ISPYS, and Tandem Basal IQ – many persons with diabetes choose to use the personalized, individual-focused therapy of DIYAPS (Braune et al., "Open-Source Automated Insulin Delivery"). It simply works well.

DIYAPS work on principles of "pay it forward" and good will. Several administrators run the Facebook group for free, which serves as a discussion group, help centre, and venting platform. In the face of the rising costs of healthcare and corporatized medicine, this could be considered a social media "miracle." If so, it is a miracle of its time. Thanks to the availability of current technology and individualized innovation, this non-hierarchical movement challenges the ways medical device companies, big pharma, doctors, and governments have traditionally controlled medical technology, medicine, and, by extension, our bodies (O'Donnell et al.). DIYAPS may revolutionize the way we treat people with diabetes and how we look at illness itself. In 2020, several manufacturers pledged to achieve interoperability among their devices. As of 2025, these promises have yet to be fulfilled. What is clear is that DIYAPS – also known as open-source artificial insulin devices (OSAID) – will be with us for a long time and have a significant effect on the medical device industry and the experience of living with diabetes.

### Phenomenological Insurrections: DIYAPS as Return to the Patient Narrative, and the Uncanny Experience of Illness

T1D is an unusual illness. The PWT1D has to navigate a multitude of decisions every day, on their own. The PWT1D tests their blood glucose, decides how much insulin to take in response to carbs ingested, and navigates factors like exercise and illness. Except for the once-every-six-months medical appointment, where a team of healthcare professionals (HCPs) review the patient's blood glucose numbers and HbA1c, it is up to the PWT1D to negotiate daily life-and-death decisions. In this sense, Loop, and the DIYAPS mentioned above, while unique from a legal, social, and economic perspective, are not a one-of-a-kind phenomenon: they are extensions of the prosthetic T1D patient experience (Matthewman 38). T1D is always a do-it-yourself affair.

While the PWT1D's experience of illness is a vital component of diabetes management, it is less prioritized in scientific literature. Relegated to the scientifically diminutive category of *qualitative analysis*, patient narratives are often considered second-class citizens when it comes to T1D research (Ritholz et al.). In this sense, philosopher Havi Carel's phenomenological argument to "return to the patient narrative" feels urgent when discussing and reflecting upon diabetes (71). Carel calls for a meaning-based approach to illness. She argues that medicine, for all its technological advancements, is limited by its biological focus on disease, creating a "measure of incommunicability" between the medical establishment and the patient's intimate understanding of themselves (46). This presents innumerable challenges from a patient's perspective when dealing with T1D, in particular when the daily experience is only superficially communicated in twice-yearly check-ups. As Hinder and Greenhalgh write, "People with diabetes spend around 1% of their time in contact with health professionals; the other 99% is virtually a closed book to clinicians and researchers" (2). Objective numbers, such as an HbA1C test, are inadequate when trying to understand a life with chronic illness, thereby falling short of engaging with what medicine ought to: healing. In our need to "return to the body" (Merleau-Ponty), Carel suggests a phenomenological approach to illness, with an emphasis on the patient experience (78). Through the countless daily decisions involved in treatment, the PWT1D is an intimate specialist of the body, offering a knowledge wrought of experience, spontaneity, and invention. Medicine needs to learn to listen to the purveyors of this knowledge.

Carel's phenomenological argument contains echoes of Rita Charon's concept of *narrative medicine*. Charon, herself a medical doctor, believes that HCPs need to "listen better" to the patient's story. She argues that medicine, in too often dismissing patient voices and assuming a paternalistic "doctor knows best" role, has limited itself in what public health can achieve and nurture; hospitals are not places of healing but confusing bureaucratic superstructures that exhaust, ignore, or condescend the patient experience (Carel 16). In Charon's view, the HCP needs to become a kind of "literary detective," decoding the narrative strands of a patient's illness story (103). While a PWT1D's illness narrative might be unreliable or inconsistent, the HCP can learn to piece together the fragments and complicated layers that chronic illness often encompasses (Charon 102).

While we agree with such improvements in medical practice and approach, the fact remains that Charon's narrative medicine is limited to the doctor's office. In the life of the PWT1D, the experience of illness occurs in the day to day. It is little surprise, then, that because of the devaluing (or ignoring) of the patient narrative in daily life, in conjunction with the revolutionary technologies now available, the chronically ill have taken matters into their own hands. Nowhere is this more apparent than with DIYAPS. Not only are the authors of this chapter members of this amorphous, transnational, Facebook-based community that refuses to wait for government legislation of new medical devices, we are alive because of it. What are the implications of a patient-driven treatment that paves the way for new therapies in the medical establishment? Are we, as Donna Haraway might intone, cyborgs of our century? If so, we are practical cyborgs, living with a host of technological intrusions, technical anomalies, and DIY hybrids (Garfinkel, "The Body-Possible"). We use the term *practical cyborg* as a counter to Haraway's nonbinary, utopian cyborg ideal, for there is little that is utopian in living with DIYAPS (Garfinkel, "The Body-Possible"). Bluetooth transmission errors, failed sensors, kinked catheters, out-of-date insulin pumps: life on Loop evokes a flawed system that requires constant maintenance and an intimate knowledge of one's technology. Yet DIYAPS are also the best artificial pancreas systems that exists. We use one because it works well, and we live better because of it (Braune et al., "Real-World Use").

The practical cyborg bends our traditional image of the narrative self in health humanities. It fills the gap in what Carel calls the neglect of the patient narrative by rewriting the PWT1D's story. This is a story that is both surprising and revolutionary, for people with diabetes, and those related to them, have used the wisdom of their experience to create a closed-loop system free for anyone to use. It is open source, bringing together a multitude of different medical devices not designed to work together, thereby challenging medical hierarchies and medical device companies' corporate focus on proprietary ambitions and biological quantities. It turns the "they" and "she" and "he" of disease into the "I" and "us" of illness (Carel 17). This journey from the objective diagnosis to one of subjective meaning is part and parcel of the DIYAPS revolution. Born of a neglect of the patient narrative, the phenomenological question then is, What is the actual experience of life with DIYAPS? Tethered to our phones, cannulas, and insulin pumps, where does the body begin and end? It is perhaps a two-way relationship, this (im)practical cyborg: as we grow into our own flesh, medical technology grows into our diabetes bodies. We become intimate with our technologies, and our technologies with us. Uncanny, perhaps – though DIYAPS also mediate and respond to the uncanny experience of living with chronic illness (Svenaeus). By removing many of the decisions and calculations (and relying on a patient-created algorithm), it lessens the burden of care. It makes the body homelike again.

In many ways, the experience of living with T1D – or any chronic illness – is an experience with the uncanny, what Heidegger called *das Unheimliche* (Svenaeus 3). Upon diagnosis, the most familiar parts of the PWT1D's life – eating, urinating, sleeping – become foreign and take on a completely new meaning. It is a difficult time that requires a network of support to make the person with diabetes's transition into a life with diabetes as smooth as possible. Doctors, nurses, specialists, and family members try to make the experience of the body – suddenly alien and uncanny because of the trauma of diagnosis – more familiar and easier to manage (Svenaeus 5). This experience of the uncanny – of this body not being quite our own – of the familiar rendered unfamiliar – doesn't ever fully disappear for the PWT1D. The chronically ill experience unhome-likeness repeatedly throughout a lifetime, our lives an oscillation between being at home in the world and the strange. In taking many of the hourly decisions out of the hands of the patient, in relieving the burden of care, DIYAPS contradictorily provide a sense of patient empowerment, as well as a sense of being more at ease in the body. We live through and intimately with our technologies.

Yet it is more than technology that helps to facilitate a sense of home-likeness. While the experience of diabetes, and any chronic illness, can feel lonely and isolating, the diabetes community – in particular, as noted, the DIYAPS community on Facebook called Looped, whose members now number in excess of 30 000 people – are a vital part of the PWT1D's well-being. Instead of a Medtronic hotline, the Looped Facebook group offers support, advice, and friendship with the click of a mouse or a tap on a device. Instead of a ten-minute visit to a doctor's office, Loopers can engage in multiple conversations with an entire community of living experts at any hour of the day in a myriad of time zones. Loopers can ask questions as they come up in real time while trying to troubleshoot life-or-death situations. As DIYAPS become more viable options for diabetes treatment (still used only among a small minority of people), there is a growing desire by the medical community to understand this patient driven treatment; healthcare professionals who want to understand how to better help their patients (Braune et al., "Open-Source Automated Insulin Delivery").

The DIYAPS community offers something vastly different from what a hospital does: a lived epistemology. Support, without the waiting times. Personalized knowledge, without bureaucracy. Workarounds, hacks, weekly software updates. This non-hierarchical, accessible, experience-based community is open to anyone with an internet connection, smartphone, CGM, and insulin pump. It suggests new ways and approaches to healthcare, or rather, redefines the notion of what living a healthy and meaningful life entails. Rather than a pass or fail report card from your doctor's office or insurance company, a conversation begins. One feels listened to. Which is a kind of healing too. But are DIYAPS truly accessible to everyone? What are the social, economic, and epistemological privileges to consider when analyzing this social movement? Is it, in fact, a social movement?

## Assessing the DIYAPS Revolution

More than ten years ago, a *British Medical Journal* (BMJ) editorial urged: "Let the patient revolution begin" (Richards et al. 346). Directed at an audience of HCPs, it sounded like a wake-up call: "Today, disease and doctor centric health systems ... are costly, wasteful, fragmented, and too often uncaring" (346). According to the authors, a key part of the solution consisted of a "fundamental shift in the power structure in healthcare" in favour of patients, with whom clinicians were called to work in closer partnership. In other words, medical paternalism had to give way to a new paradigm putting patients first, both as moral and epistemic agents: "Healthcare won't get better until patients play a leading role in fixing it" the editorial concluded, meaning not only that patients' personal values and preferences had to be respected but also that their unique perspective on their conditions, needs, and appropriate ways to address them had to be duly taken into account (Richards et al. 347).

As radical as it looked *prima facie*, this injunction may also have seemed like a damp squib for many patients and their representatives, as this so-called "revolution" had already begun well before 2013. It hit the public's attention during the infamous HIV epidemics back in the 1980s, especially through ACT UP protests and disruptive interventions. Catchy slogans like "Knowledge is power," "Silence = death," or "Nothing about us without us" became popular and have remained highly influential ever since, including for PWT1D advocacy groups (Irwin).

The striking mismatch between what the BMJ's editorial entailed – a pending revolution – and what was already happening on the ground according to activists themselves is hardly surprising. As urgent or recurrent as it may be, addressing the needs of a particular sub-group of the population on an institutional level takes time. Often, it is the less than perfect result of a long and strenuous negotiation process between stakeholders and institutions whose agendas and values diverge (e.g., intervention's efficiency versus safety). Success is never guaranteed. In this section, we attempt to situate the DIYAPS initiative as it is trying to make its way through this process.

DIYAPS development and diffusion epitomize patients' empowerment and autonomy at its highest, and they are adequately portrayed as such in nearly every scientific paper. As mentioned, it sprang from an earlier initiative that was primarily concerned with transparency and access to health data: the #WeAreNotWaiting movement. According to Timothy Omer, a long-standing patients' advocate and self-identified activist, the DIYAPS initiative resulted from the conjunction of two independent trends in health-related technology: on the one hand, the commercialization of CGM, and on the other hand, the rise of social media and development of one-line communities, providing patients with a platform not only for mutual support but also for information dissemination and lively debates about existing diabetes-related technologies. Common frustrations and unmet needs were articulated. But things did not stop there; quite the contrary: projects and action plans were quickly also laid out. As Omer puts it, "the community declared 'We are not waiting.' And rightly so, why should patients wait to address their current needs?" (118). Thus, it is unquestionable that DIYAPS, as a patient-driven project that involves elements of biohacking and innovation, which outpaced industrials and researchers, are revolutionary. They set a striking example of what patients, or at least some of them, are capable of. They have quickly drawn social scientists' attention, and a growing literature is now dedicated to scrutinizing their ins and outs in the context of personalized and technology mediated healthcare. The DIYAPS user (or Looper) is an outstanding specimen of what "patient 2.0" and "eHealth" are supposed to look like and can provide valuable insights about how the future of healthcare and public involvement could take shape in the foreseeable future (Gaddi et al.).

However, there might be an overlooked flip side to that coin. First, even though the DIYAPS initiative aims at providing the best treatment options to the greatest number of people in the most cost-effective way (hence the open-source and not-for-profit nature of the whole project), its accessibility still heavily relies on socio-economic factors, starting with the kind of public healthcare and more generally the resources (including time) people can invest in it. Now, 100 years after insulin was discovered and despite its inscription on the World Health Organization's essential medicines list in 1977, it is estimated that 50 percent of people around the world in need of insulin (including both PWT1D and those with type 2 diabetes) cannot reliably access it because it is unavailable and/or unaffordable (World Health Organization). Even in high-income countries like the United States, an alarming number of patients have to ration their insulin because of its skyrocketing costs (Fralick and Kesselheim).[1] Scholars readily acknowledge that "engaging

1 It is not easy to assess the financial burden living with type 1 diabetes represents, even in Canada. According to a Diabetes Canada report issued in 2023 costs vary greatly depending on each province and territories' public insurance programs. Public coverage ranges from 100 percent to 0 percent depending on age, location, and income. For instance, insulin pumps are covered for both children and adults in some provinces, but only for children under 18 in others. Family income is also a major factor. Thus in 2022, a PWT1D under 18 living in a household with an income of CAD 30 000/year paid around CAD 78 out of pocket in Alberta for their CGM and insulin pump. By contrast, someone of the same age living in a high-income household (CAD 150 000 and above) had to pay 18 306 CAD in New Brunswick for identical devices. In Quebec, people over 65 earning CAD 30 000 or less per year devoted up to 20 percent of their income to accessing these medical devices and supplies. To sum up: T1D is an expensive chronic disease to live with that can take a significant toll on both public and personal finances. Even though people can live with the disease without resorting to technologies like CGM and insulin pumps and stick to multiple daily injections and capillary blood testing (which some people prefer: some don't feel comfortable continuously wearing visible devices on their bodies; others do not trust technology or are bothered by the various alarms or have concerns about their private health data

in this practice ['closing the loop'] demands a lot of determination and mobilization of social and material resources" (Jansky and Langstrup 501), but the socio-demographic data of participants in most qualitative studies are strikingly homogeneous: on average, DIYAPS users interviewed are middle-age, disproportionately white, employed, and educated. A recent paper reporting the results of the first large scale survey on adults with T1D and caregivers using DIYAPS (897 people from over 35 countries) showed that 77 percent of participants were from Europe, 14 percent from North America, and only 9 percent from "other continents" (Braune et al., "Why #WeAreNotWaiting"). Among adults living with T1D, almost 83 percent (and over 87 percent among caregivers) had a university degree or higher (12.4 percent had a doctorate). Finally, 57.2 percent of participants had a household annual net income of USD 50,000 or higher (21.2 percent over USD 100 000). As wide and varied as it was, this sample is obviously non representative of the PWT1D population around the world. Even though the authors acknowledge potential recruitment bias, these numbers should give us pause, as published papers both in clinical medicine and the social sciences may give the impression that DIYAPS are more widely accessible and used than they actually are. Especially in the context of the so-called "insulin crisis," which hits people from both the United States and many non-western countries, DIYAPS is not even remotely an option. If anything, it is a revolution for the most privileged.

Other concerns are the moral and social features that tend to be associated with Loopers in the media and through social networks: the public figure of the DIY Looper has so far been one of moral rectitude (caring parents – so-called "D-dads"– or spouses, patients committed to sharing and supporting each other, eager to "give back to the community") and intellectually gifted (clever, pragmatic, innovative, able to think outside the box, ingenious, etc.) (Kesavadev et al.). In that respect, they perfectly fit a long-standing stereotype attached to PWT1D: the

---

being hacked or shared with third parties, etc.), they are considered the gold standard for T1D treatment according to most national clinical practice guidelines. So, for reasons as random as the region a person lives in or at what age they were diagnosed, access to the very treatment recommended by physicians may be hindered, even in a wealthy country such as Canada whose health system remains mostly public. Injustices plaguing PWT1D are all the more blatant when the issue of treatment availability and affordability is viewed from a more global perspective. According to T1 International, a non-profit organization led by people with T1D working to improve access to treatment worldwide, 50 percent of people in need of insulin could not reliably access it in 2015 because it was unavailable, unaffordable, or both. Without insulin, the life expectancy of a PWT1D is a couple of months, at best.

"good citizen."[2] Current literature on the "supercrip athlete" stereotype may be relevant here: supercrip athletes are "those individuals whose inspirational stories of courage, dedication, and hard work prove that it can be done, that one can defy the odds and accomplish the impossible" (Berger 647). While their spectacular achievements may contribute to debunking prejudices and stigma against people living with an impairment, it has also been argued that their doing so may enforce and validate ableist criteria of success,[3] and mistakenly put the emphasis on individual moral virtues like courage, commitment, perseverance, or grit, whereas the external and socio-economic factors that contributed to their success remain unaccounted for. Certainly, by building their own DIYAPS and optimizing their treatment so that it fits their individual needs better than any commercial system on the market could ever do, a Looper outsmarts anyone else: other patients and HCPs as well. So far, the health-related outcomes they achieve turn out to be nothing short of spectacular, at least in terms of health related outcomes and experiences (quality of sleep, cognitive and emotional burden, perceived safety, and quality of life in general).[4] Thus, it is tempting to portray Loopers as some kind of elite, super-patients who successfully took matters into their own hands, reverse-engineered commercial devices, hacked pumps, and coded algorithms, while being eager to share and teach their skills to whoever needs it. Especially on social media, they can look like – and sometimes self-advocate as – some extraordinary mix of top scientists, engineers, educators, and cyborg/mutant vigilantes serving their community's greater good. A recent study on social-media-driven health movements, especially on Twitter (now X), came up with a cartography of the different types of users' "personas" in order to "understand the 'type' of person who engaged, amplified, and drove the #WeAreNotWaiting and #OpenAPS conversation," using discourse analysis (Lichtman et al.). The authors list six main categories, the first four being labelled "fearless leaders," "loopers living it up,"

2 This stereotype relies on the assumption that because T1D treatment requires relentless self-management, self-control, and moderation (especially in food intake), PWT1D have virtually no other choice except to acquire these virtues. The contrast with type 2 diabetes is striking, as people living with type 2 diabetes are usually seen as overweight, self-indulgent, weak or irresponsible (see Tuchman).

3 T1D has supercrip athletes of its own, including Sébastien Sasseville, a PWT1D and self-professed "motivational speaker" who climbed Mount Everest and completed six Ironman Triathlons. Elite hockey player Max Domi is also a public T1D figure, sponsored by various medical device companies including Medtronic.

4 The lack of robust data and of studies meeting the standards of evidence-based medicine is at the heart of the concerns for most healthcare providers. (See Shepard et al.)

"parents on a mission," and "tech titans." This wording enforces the impression that most people engaged in the DIYAPS conversation are super- (self-) empowered patients who may contribute to "think and create differently regarding personal healthcare and somatic issues" as they "take means of production into their own hands and thus challenge production and knowledge practices in biomedicine" (Jansky and Langstrup 508). They also appear as morally superior since they share a pay-it-forward ethos, showing how "the innovation of the closed-loop system only exists if you make it possible for others" (Jansky and Langstrup 516).

Thus, once again: although the #WeAreNotWaiting movement and DIYAPS initiative exemplify genuine revolutionary features and involve some truly exceptional characters, their political and social outreach should be cautiously assessed. As Gottlieb rightly points out:

> Although the PWT1D communities who have designed and built their own systems are exceptionally motivated and effective, their efforts do not solve the many inequities in T1D disease management, especially in the US. Open sources solutions have yet to solve the high cost of insulin and the uneven access to T1D technologies. ... these issues of access and cost lurk as problems that must be solved through policy and regulatory interventions rather than patients incurring the burden of "empowerment" to solve a problem that individuals cannot directly impact. (210)

Our intention is neither to downplay the width and significance of the DIYAPS initiative, nor to question the morality of its promoters' intentions. If anything, they deserve praise and admiration. On the other hand, especially as social scientists, one should resist the temptation to over-romanticize this "patients' revolution" and obtain some perspective on its wider social and political aspects.[5]

---

5 Here, a critical stance could be adopted towards the whole DIYAPS movement, especially when undertaking to account for its emergence and significance through the lens of contemporary critical studies on digital health. On the one hand, the "pay it forward" ethos that drives the work and efforts of most of the participants involved in this initiative is unquestionable, and as far as we can tell, it has helped and empowered people by the thousands. On the other hand, it is also likely to reproduce and reinforce certain assumptions about health, (dis-)abled bodies, and technologies' benefits, which could and probably should be challenged. Because of a lack of empirical data and because what we are dealing with here is a phenomenon whose shape, evolution, and outreach are still largely unknown, we feel that it is premature to draw any sort of normative or substantial conclusions. However, the insightful work of scholars like Olivia Banner provides a helpful critical framework to look at

## DIYAPS: Navigating Risks and Fostering Alliance

In a very weak sense, any do-it-yourself project does involve some sort of activism, as DIYers actively engage in the production of the goods they intend to consume, rather than passively buying and using standardized, industrially ready-made devices. Since in our case, the product is a life-sustaining device, it is reasonable to assume that opting for a DIYAPS is the outcome of a careful process of deliberation and assessment of the risks-benefits balance. Even though people engaging in DIYAPS are generally among the most privileged in terms of socio-demographic features, doing so remains risky, and this is made very clear by its promoters online: they inform the user that it is an experimental patient-led initiative, endorsed neither by public health authorities nor device manufacturers, in which people engage ultimately at their own risk. However, DIYAPS as such are not illegal. True, it would not have been possible if not for Ben West's discovery and active exploitation of a security failure of his insulin pump, thus a genuine act of biohacking. On the other hand, the greater control over an insulin-delivering device gained that way hardly amounts to diverting the technology: rather, "closing the loop" results in it fulfilling the exact function it was designed to perform. It is not hijacked, since Loopers are its rightful owners; neither is it misused. On the contrary, it is improved and enhanced to the limits of its possibilities. Thus, an otherwise industrial one-size-fits-all product is turned into a highly personal, tailor-made, and better performing system.

True, insulin is a powerful medication. Administration and/or titration errors can lead to dramatic and life-threatening consequences, and a recent study suggests that insulin overdosing is likely to be used in the context of suicide or self-injury attempts by PWT1D (Barnard-Kelly et al.). But we should resist hasty conclusions when it comes to the risk of patients abusing or misusing insulin, be it deliberate or accidental. The very nature of T1D management as it has been generally promoted and implemented, hopefully for the best, by HCPs and patients' representatives is that of an autonomous daily self-care practice. To the extent that it encompasses not only clinical interventions (blood glucose testing, insulin administration) but also the management of food intake

---

the DIYAPS initiative and how it is unfolding as it makes its way to more corporate, mainstream markets thanks to the health regulation by federal health authorities (see, for instance, the Tidepool-Loop project, a mobile app that was approved by the FDA just as this chapter was being written: https://www.tidepool.org/tidepool-loop). We thank our reviewers for drawing our attention to these points.

and physical activity, and impacts virtually every dimension of a person's life (cognitions as well as emotions, work, family, social relationships, and so on), it can almost be seen as a way of life of its own. As a means of managing T1D people may choose to adopt with or without medical supervision, DIYAPS is congenial and part of a lot of other self-care behaviours: for instance, engaging in a low-carb diet, alternating high- and low-impact exercise routines, meditating, and so forth. Whereas physicians may worry about their patients relying on self-medicating practices, especially over-the-counter medication and so-called complementary and alternative medicines, the epistemic stance towards biomedicine exemplified by the DIYAPS community is one characterized by informed trust and reliance: the current scientific and clinical views about how to explain and manage T1D are taken for granted and presumed accurate, rather than questioned. On the contrary, DIYAPS are hardly for beginners (Davis): candidates need to be "type 1 diabetes-literate," if not actual (lay-)experts, since they have to be familiar with CGM and insulin pump use already, as well as being able to understand and use a vast array of technical concepts that only diabetes educators and endocrinologists would share (e.g., *insulin on board*, *basal rate*, *dawn phenomenon*). In that respect, their knowledge and skills do not compete with but encompass and extend that of HCPs.

This results in a striking epistemic shift in the clinical encounter: DIYAPS is a patient-led initiative for which, things being as they are, HCPs are not and cannot be trained. There are at least two reasons at play here: first, DIYAPS is not endorsed by regulatory institutions, exposing them to liability and ethical issues; second, their training and certification for using a new medical device or treatment regimen is the exclusive domain of pharmaceutical companies and their representatives. This means that learning about DIYAPS is a matter of personal choice: it doesn't yet pertain to the list of accredited continuing professional development activities and ought to be done in off-work hours. Thus, it is even more admirable that, though still marginal, a growing community of HCPs is now siding with their patients who decided to resort to DIYAPS as part of their duty of care and are proactively collecting suitable information to help them do so in the most accurate and safe way (Wu et al.). While a few of them even go as far as arguing in favour of DIYAPS prescription, most rather insist that its benefits and safety are worthy of a systematic re-evaluation in terms of outcomes and safety compared to commercial systems (Braune et al., "Open-Source Automated Insulin Delivery"). While several studies have already been realized, most of them are deemed of low significance because they do not meet the usual standards of evidence-based medicine and rely on observational, retrospective, and/or patient-reported data. DIYAPS stand consistently acknowledged as a promising avenue for T1D management nevertheless (Jennings and Hussain).

In many respects, it seems that the DIYAPS revolution is on the verge of fulfilling all its promises, in terms of both health-related and political outcomes. If its efficiency and safety were to be firmly established once and for all, it would provide a striking proof that sanitary democracy is achievable, a system in which citizen-patients are genuine partners in healthcare and positively contribute to the improvement of public health (Burnside et al.). As we have seen, numerous obstacles, both epistemic, social, and political, have arguably been successfully overcome, defying the odds. How so? This should, and will most probably, be scrutinized in future studies. For the time being, it is reasonable to hypothesize that the DIYAPS movement has gained traction mostly because it has been developed by people either living with T1D or caring for someone who does. Obviously, this has largely contributed to fostering a sense of reassurance, belonging, and trust in other patients, in a context where pharmaceutical companies have been criticized for their greediness and indifference towards their consumers' well-being. By contrast, DIYAPS enjoy the reputation of benevolence attached to local, horizontal, DIY, and community-based initiatives. Besides, it hinges upon, rather than challenges, current biomedical knowledge. Patients' trust would have easily been lost if significant accidents or adverse effects had been reported. But so far, there are more deaths and health-related incidents, especially diabetes-related ketoacidosis, that are due to insulin rationing than to DIYAPS use (Herkert et al.).

A second, closely related, key element is the remarkable investment that has been made by DIYAPS leaders and promoters to reach and support other PWT1D. Once again, their praiseworthy commitment to improving the community's wellness and extend treatment options should not be undervalued. It is a not-for-profit initiative, primarily based on altruistic motives and guided by democratic values like openness, shareability, knowledge dissemination, and peer support. Especially striking is the breadth of work they are dedicating to render DIYAPS accessible to non-tech-savvy people. Building an app, running diagnostics, and troubleshooting are operations that most laypeople would understandingly find impressive, overly complex, unachievable, or just annoying and time consuming. Remarkable resources have been devoted to help overcome these various obstacles: in particular, a step-by-step guide detailing every part of the system's implementation (or "building") process is available. It is written in lay English, with a profusion of screens shots and links to video tutorials, and a realistic estimate of the required time to complete each step. On social media, some groups provide mentorships and organize one-line as well as in-person so-called "building parties," where advanced users supervise and help newcomers. Thus, risks are mitigated, but of course problems and drawbacks happen: for instance, most DIYAPS apps run on cellphones and tablets, whose operating systems are continually updated by companies' developers without any consideration for off-label apps. Therefore, it is crucial for DIYAPS users to stay tuned and wait for the community's green light before installing any OS update. Disabling automatic updates is highly recommended, with the ensuing impediments this may involve. Transmission loss and connectivity failure may also occur in certain circumstances, requiring the user to react promptly and activate various troubleshooting skills, resources, and autonomy.

Overall, the DIYAPS community encompasses various types of members, some of whom would hardly self-identify as health activists, let alone biohackers. As social scientists working on DIY communities have emphasized, turning to a do-it-yourself technology is foremost a consumer behaviour. While "the consumer typically is viewed only as the passive buyer of what others produce and not as the active producer of goods or services," people resorting to DIY projects fall rather under the umbrella of "prosumers" – namely, "consumers producing products for their own consumption," being both the designers of the functional specifications and their builder (Wolf and McQuitty 154). According to Wolf and McQuitty, "they choose among available materials and tools, engineer the work process to complete the project, and act as inspectors and evaluators when deciding whether the product has achieved the desired value," DIY projects being typically labour-intensive (154). Coined by Alvin Toffler, the label *prosumer* refers to people playing both the role of consumers and (co-)producers, the latter referring to the fact that they endorse tasks that would traditionally be overseen by company employees. As they start looping, PWT1D simultaneously do what, in other circumstances, pharmaceutical companies R&D departments and/or healthcare providers would do or provide (technological means and personalized settings). The term *prosumer* is useful because it captures the diversity of motivations that can lead a given individual to use a DIYAPS: whereas some people engage in such projects as a concrete way to resist consumerism, industrial monopolies, and capitalist ideology at large, some do so out of mere curiosity, while others do it for personal convenience. As within other tech-oriented DIY groups, a majority of the DIYAPS community members are probably rather on the receiving, user, or consumer end, than on the conception, engineering, and/or production end. Especially as it is reaching momentum and success, DIYAPS may lose part of their activism flavour and impetus. Whether or not it will keep its traction once industrials will be able to meet the demand of their customers for more effective and personalized treatment options remains an open question.

## Conclusion

In this chapter, we attempted to unfold the various perspectives (personal, phenomenological, moral, social, and political) from which the DIYAPS movement may be suitably apprehended. Because it started only a little over ten years ago, it would certainly be premature to claim that we achieved to establish anything definitive: much of the science, so to say, remains undone. Considering the remarkable amount of attention such a disruptive patient-driven initiative has already managed to draw to itself, there is every reason to think that it will continue to be scrutinized and that fruitful discussions will ensue. For the time being, DIYAPS appears as a decisive milestone in the history of healthcare democratization and patient empowerment in the twenty-first century. While it may be viewed as delivering a long-awaited coup de grâce to paternalism in doctor-patient relationships, it also leads us to reassess the foundations and aims of care. If anything, DIYAPS users are what some patient-education programs have long strived to bring about: an ideal community of educated, skilled, motivated, and self-reliant individuals – in other words, patients who could almost do without doctors. But our concerns here are not only about PWT1D learning to live well outside the institutional and hierarchical constraints of the healthcare profession. Rather, we believe that DIYAPS has the potential to contribute to an evolving relationship between patients and HCPs. Perhaps, in reflecting on the disjunct between the first-person patient narrative and third-person physician perspectives, there may emerge what Havi Carel calls a second-person point of view (47). In other words: empathy and understanding. It is not always clear whether HCPs *prima facie* defiance towards DIYAPS is grounded in sheer ethical and medico-legal concerns (Burnside et al. 880) or rather motivated by ignorance, prejudice, and the fear of losing their authority and power over their patients. In the latter case at least, we hope that in the future HCPs will move past these inhibitions. For when a HCP tries to understand the patient's lived experience, approaching DIYAPS with both curiosity and the humility to learn and learn better, they also learn to listen. And the patient, empowered by their own peculiar, flawed story, begins to tell it, learning new truths as they tell, retell, and edit along the way.

We say this with the humility of knowing that as efficient and safe as they may be, DIYAPS, whatever their future, are but a means to manage T1D, not a cure: even "expert-patients" have to navigate the uncertainties associated with living with a chronic condition whose course over time remains unpredictable, especially as they age, a prosthetic living we cannot do alone.

## WORKS CITED

Banner, O. *Communicative Biocapitalism: The Voice of the Patient in Digital Health and the Health Humanities*. U of Michigan P, 2017.

Barnard-Kelly, K. D., et al. "An Intolerable Burden: Suicide, Intended Self-Injury and Diabetes." *Canadian Journal of Diabetes*, vol. 44, no. 6, 2020, pp. 541–44, https://doi.org/10.1016/j.jcjd.2020.01.008.

Berger, R. J. "Disability and the Dedicated Wheelchair Athlete: Beyond the 'Supercrip' critique." *Journal of Contemporary Ethnography*, vol. 37, no. 6, 2008, pp. 647–78, https://doi.org/10.1177/0891241607309892.

Braune, K., et al. "Real-World Use of Do-It-Yourself Artificial Pancreas Systems in Children and Adolescents with Type 1 Diabetes: Online Survey and Analysis of Self-Reported Clinical Outcomes." *JMIR mHealth and uHealth*, vol. 7, no. 7, 2019, Article e14087, http://mhealth.jmir.org/2019/7/e14087/.

–. "Open-Source Automated Insulin Delivery: International Consensus Statement and Practical Guidance for Health-Care Professionals." *Lancet Diabetes Endocrinology*, vol. 10, 2021, p. 63, https://doi.org/10.10/16/S2213-8587(21)00267-9.

–. "Why #WeAreNotWaiting – Motivations and Self-Reported Outcomes Among Users of Open-Source Automated Insulin Delivery Systems: Multinational Survey." *Journal of Medical Internet Research*, vol. 23, no. 6, 2021, Article e25409, https://doi.org/10.2196/25409.

Burnside, M., et al. "Do-It-Yourself Automated Insulin Delivery: A Leading Example of the Democratization of Medicine." *Journal of Diabetes Science and Technology*, vol. 14, no. 5, 2020, pp. 878–82, https://doi.org/10.1177/1932296819890623.

Carel, Havi. *Phenomenology of Illness*. Oxford UP, 2016.

Charon, Rita. *Narrative Medicine: Honoring the Stories of Illness*. Oxford UP, 2006.

Cleal, B., et al. "Living on the Loop – Agency, Skill and (Re)enchantment in DIY Artificial Pancreas System Use," 2021, http://francisconunes.me/RealizingAIinHealthcareWS/papers/Cleal2021.pdf.

Davis, Clay. "The Routinization of Lay Expertise: A Diachronic Account of the Invention and Stabilization of an Open-Source Artificial Pancreas." *Social Studies of Science*, vol. 54, no. 4, 2024, pp. 626–52.

Diabetes Canada. "Diabetes and Diabetes-Related Out-of-Pocket Costs: 2022 Update." *Diabetes Canada*, 2023. https://www.diabetes.ca/DiabetesCanadaWebsite/media/Advocacy-and-Policy/Advocacy%20Reports/Diabetes-Canada-2022-Out-Of-Pocket-Report-EN-FINAL.pdf.

Feudtner, Chris. *Bittersweet: Diabetes, Insulin and the Transformation of Illness*. U of North Carolina P, 2003.

Fralick, M., and A. S. Kesselheim. "The U.S. Insulin Crisis – Rationing a Lifesaving Medication Discovered in the 1920s." *New England Journal of Medicine*, vol. 381, no. 19, 2019, pp. 1793–95, https://doi.org/10.1056/NEJMp1909402.

Gaddi, Antonio, et al. *eHealth, Care and Quality of Life*, Springer, 2013. https://doi.org/10.1007/978-88-470-5253-6.

Garfinkel, Jonathan. "Hacking Diabetes." *Walrus Magazine*, Jan. 2020. https://thewalrus.ca/hacking-diabetes/.

–. "The Body-Possible and Practical Cyborg: Isabelle Van Grimde's *Eve 2050*." *Dyscorpia: Intersections of the Body and Technology*, Art exhibition catalogue. U of Alberta P, 2020, pp. 62–73.

Gottlieb, S. D. "The Fantastical Empowered Patient." *Healthcare Activism: Markets, Morals, and the Collective Good*, edited by Susi Geiger, Oxford UP, 2021. pp. 198–223.

Gottlieb, S. D., and J. Cluck. "'Going Rogue': Re-coding Resistance with Type 1 Diabetes." *Digital Culture & Society*, vol. 4, no. 2, 2018, pp. 43–44, https://doi.org/10.14361/dcs-2018-0208.

Haraway, Donna. *A Cyborg Manifesto*. U of Minnesota P, 2016.

Herkert, D., et al. "Cost-Related Insulin Underuse Among Patients With Diabetes." *JAMA Internal Medicine*, vol. 179, no. 1, 2019, pp. 112–14, https://doi.org/10.1001/jamainternmed.2018.5008.

Hinder, S., and T. Greenhalgh. "'This Does My Head In': Ethnographic Study of Self-Management by People with Diabetes." *BMC Health Services Research*, vol. 12, no. 83, 2012, pp. 1–16, https://doi.org/10.1186/1472-6963-12-83.

Irwin, Clair. "The #insulin4all Movement: A Few Committed Individuals Isn't Enough." *(Un)doing Diabetes: Representation, Disability, Culture*, edited by C. C. Frazer and H. R. Walker, Palgrave, 2021, pp. 63–82.

Jansky, B., and H. Langstrup. "Device Activism and Material Participation in Healthcare: Retracing Forms of Engagement in the #WeAreNotWaiting Movement for Open-Source Closed-Loop Systems in Type 1 Diabetes Self-Care." *BioSocieties*, vol. 18, 2023, pp. 498–522, https://doi.org/10.1057/s41292-022-00278-4.

Jennings P., and S. Hussain. "Do-It-Yourself Artificial Pancreas Systems: A Review of the Emerging Evidence and Insights for Healthcare Professionals." *Journal of Diabetes Science and Technology*, vol. 14, no. 5, 2020, pp. 868–77, https://doi.org/10.1177/1932296819894296.

Kesavadev, J., et al. "The Do-It-Yourself Artificial Pancreas: A Comprehensive Review." *Diabetes Therapy*, vol. 11, no. 6, 2020, pp. 1217–35. https://doi.org/10.1007/s13300-020-00823-z.

Lee, J. M., et al. "A Patient-Designed Do-It-Yourself Mobile Technology System for Diabetes: Promise and Challenges for a New Era in Medicine." *JAMA*, vol. 315, no. 14, 2016, pp. 1447–48.

Lichtman, M. L., et al. "Patient-Driven Diabetes Technologies: Sentiment and Personas of the #WeAreNotWaiting and #OpenAPS Movements." *Journal of Diabetes Science and Technology*, vol. 14, no. 6, 2020, pp. 990–99, https://doi.org/10.1177/1932296820932928.

Liu, Shengxin, et al. "Association and Familial Coaggregation of Childhood-Onset Type 1 Diabetes With Depression, Anxiety, and Stress-Related Disorders: A Population-Based Cohort Study." *Diabetes Care*, vol. 45, no. 9, 2022, pp. 1987–93, https://doi.org/10.2337/dc21-1347.

Matthewman, S. "Theorising Personal Medical Devices." *Quantified Lives and Vital Data*. Palgrave Macmillan, 2018.

Merleau-Ponty, Maurice. *The Phenomenology of Perception.* Routledge, 1994.

O'Donnell, Shane, et al. "Evidence on User-Led Innovation in Diabetes Technology (The OPEN Project): Protocol for a Mixed Methods Study." *MIR Res Protocols*, vol. 8, no. 11, 2019, Article e15368, http://www.researchprotocols.org/2019/11/e15368/.

Omer, Timothy. "Empowered Citizen 'Health Hackers' Who Are Not Waiting." *BMC Medicine*, vol. 14, no. 118, 2016, https://doi.org/10.1186/s12916-016-0670-y.

Richards Tessa, et al. "Let the Patient Revolution Begin." *British Medical Journal*, vol. 346, 2013, Article f2614, https://doi.org/10.1136/bmj.f2614.

Ritholz, Marilyn D., et al. "Digging Deeper: The Role of Qualitative Research in Behavioral Diabetes." *Current Diabetes Representations*, vol. 11, 2011, pp. 494–502, https://doi.org/10.1007/s11892-011-0226-7.

Shepard, J. A., et al. "User and Healthcare Professional Perspectives on Do-It-Yourself Artificial Pancreas Systems: A Need for Guidelines." *Journal of Diabetes Science and Technology*, vol. 16, no. 1, 2022, pp. 224–27. https://doi.org/10.1177/1932296820957728.

Svenaeus, Frederick. "Das unheimliche – Towards a Phenomenology of Illness." *Medicine, Health Care and Philosophy*, vol. 3, 2000, pp. 3–16, https://doi.org/10.1023/a:1009943524301. Medline:11080964.

Toffler, A. *The Third Wave*. William Morrow and Company Inc, 1980.

Tuchman, Arleen M. *Diabetes: A History of Race and Disease*. Yale UP, 2020.

Wolf, M., and S. McQuitty. "Understanding the Do-It-Yourself Consumer: DIY Motivations and Outcomes." *AMS Review*, vol. 1, 2011, pp. 154–70, https://doi.org/10.1007/s13162-011-0021-2.

World Health Organization. "WHO Launches First-Ever Insulin Prequalification Program to Expand Access to Life-Saving Treatment for

Diabetes." *World Health Organization*, 13 Nov. 2019, https://www.who.int/news/item/13-11-2019-who-launches-first-ever-insulin-prequalification-programme-to-expand-access-to-life-saving-treatment-for-diabetes.

Wu, Z., et al. "Use of a Do-It-Yourself Artificial Pancreas System Is Associated with Better Glucose Management and Higher Quality of Life among Adults with Type 1 Diabetes." *Therapeutic Advances in Endocrinology and Metabolism*, vol. 11, 2020. https://doi.org/10.1177/2042018820950146.

# 9 Embodied Books: Sensing Healthcare Experiences in Artists' Books

DARIAN GOLDIN STAHL

Books have been mobilized to hold, archive, and disseminate patient voices for centuries, but what about the healthcare experiences that elude words? Even the addition of images and photographs might fail to capture what it is like to live daily with a life-altering diagnosis or impending mortality. Physical barriers to writing a comprehensible narrative or lacking the capital and connections to publish books further inhibit the breadth of healthcare experiences readers and researchers can access. In short, whose stories are not included in the literary canon of health humanities because they cannot be written?

I argue that the hybrid medium of art and book object, known as the *artist's book*, is an accessible and more holistic format to capture expressions of health and illness than writing is capable of alone. The possibility of including a vast variety of artistic modes like drawing, painting, printmaking, photography, collage, sewing, and even performance, while also retaining the book object's capacities for archiving and dissemination, provides the author-makers with myriad possibilities to make themselves understood. The activation of the senses while engaging with the artist's book produces additional layered and embodied strategies to build intersubjectivity. Finally, I assert that artists' books have untapped potential within health education not only to expose learners to a broader range of first-person, primary experiences of medicine and illness but also in their ability to foster and sustain empathy.

To get these creative and underrepresented stories of illness in front of healthcare learners, I developed a two-part project for my Social Sciences and Humanities Research Council of Canada Banting Postdoctoral Fellowship at the University of Northern British Columbia's Northern Medical Program and Health Arts Research Centre, *Embodied Books: Binding Together Illness, Art, and Learning*. The first step of the project is to facilitate the creation of new artists' books with diverse groups of participants who want to express their lived experiences of illness, disability, caretaking, and navigating healthcare systems. The second step is to archive and disseminate these creations where they may be incorporated into medical humanities curricula. Although there are notable (albeit few) artist's book collections that are currently being mobilized within medical humanities pedagogies in the United States (Tuttle and Miller) and UK (Bolaki and Ciricaite), *Embodied Books* is the first of its kind in Canada and unique in its outreach to intrepid makers who may have never even heard of artists' books before, much less have an established artist's book practice, to take up this medium and explore the possibilities of its format to communicate their medical experiences.

I believe there is no other medium that can sensorially communicate the bodily impacts of illness and medicine quite like artists' books. This medium, at a fundamental level, is an activation of bodies. Unlike viewing art on a wall or a performance on stage, artists' books are an invitation to touch. Holding them close to the body, feeling their weight in your hands, and exploring the textural surface with your fingertips demonstrates how embodied and interactive an artist's book can truly be. Further, the multi-sensory interactions of touch, sight, scent, the performative gesture of turning pages, and spending time with the book object in an intimate one-on-one encounter makes this art form a powerhouse of phenomenological connection that can hardly be matched by any other medium.

My first artist's book was an attempt to understand another person's body better – that of my sister, Dr. Devan Stahl, who is a medical ethicist at Baylor University and was diagnosed with multiple sclerosis in 2008. Because I found myself incapable of putting words to what I wanted to express after her diagnosis and initial years of treatment, I began making artists' books with and about my sister as a way to *show* her my care and empathy. I used the skills I had acquired as a printmaker and bookmaker to layer her MRI scans with her own illness narratives so that Devan might reclaim some control over the medicalized images of her body and, ultimately, aid in the cultivation of meaning for her illness.

After developing an artist's book practice with Devan, I wondered if others might also benefit from making artists' books about their illnesses. Might they learn something more or different about their own lived experiences by structuring them across the pages of the book? And how might the sensory aspects of artists' books enable new expressive languages to arise? Finally, I wondered what value may be generated by sharing this artistic material with medical professionals and students. Thus, the *Embodied Books* project was born. The remainder of this paper explores the communication strategies of individual creations, intersubjectivity of group readings and interpretations, and the books' potential to impact medical humanities research and pedagogy.

## Sensory Communication

So far, I have conducted two five-week long artist's book courses with a total of nineteen participants who identify as being ill, disabled, and/or familial caretakers. One of these courses was held in person in the fall of 2021 at the Two Rivers Gallery in Prince George, British Columbia, and the other was held remotely online in the winter of 2022 in order to be inclusive and accessible to those who were unable to meet in person. I provided the participants with the materials, knowhow, and creative prompts to craft two or three distinct artists' books based on their lived experiences navigating healthcare systems and daily life with illness.

In addition to expressive combinations of text and image, which are thoroughly explored in many other forms of autobiographical narratives on healthcare like memoirs, graphic medicine, and illness comics, the ability to craft a book from scratch enabled new creative possibilities for structure, interaction, and materiality in print media. A particularly salient urge from the participants was to transform the typical codex book format into an abstract model of their bodies. For example, one participant rounded his book's edges and splayed open the pages to mimic the form of a three-dimensional brain, and instead of using words to express the feeling of his seizures, he used progressively intensifying shades of colour and texture to communicate their waves of magnitude – all bound together under an undulating belt of leather (see Figure 9.1).

As he is incapable of formulating words during his frequent seizures, it felt right for this maker to express his illness in the absence of text. Additionally, the "reading in the round" aspect of this book's sculptural format indicates that there is no end to this illness, only periods of rest and intensity. The structure and materiality of his book wordlessly communicate the chronic aspects of this participant's diagnosis.

Perhaps this transference of body to book is not surprising. In addition to activating the body while reading, the book form itself has parallel corporeal structures. Books contain a face, back, and spine, and we cover them in leather skins or place them within jackets to keep them protected. The commonplace metaphors of identity, thoughts, and histories being *written on the flesh* or being able to *read someone like a book* further connect the notions of book and body. If the goal is to express some ineffable aspect of one's illness or disability, transforming the book into a navigable body is a clever strategy to do so.

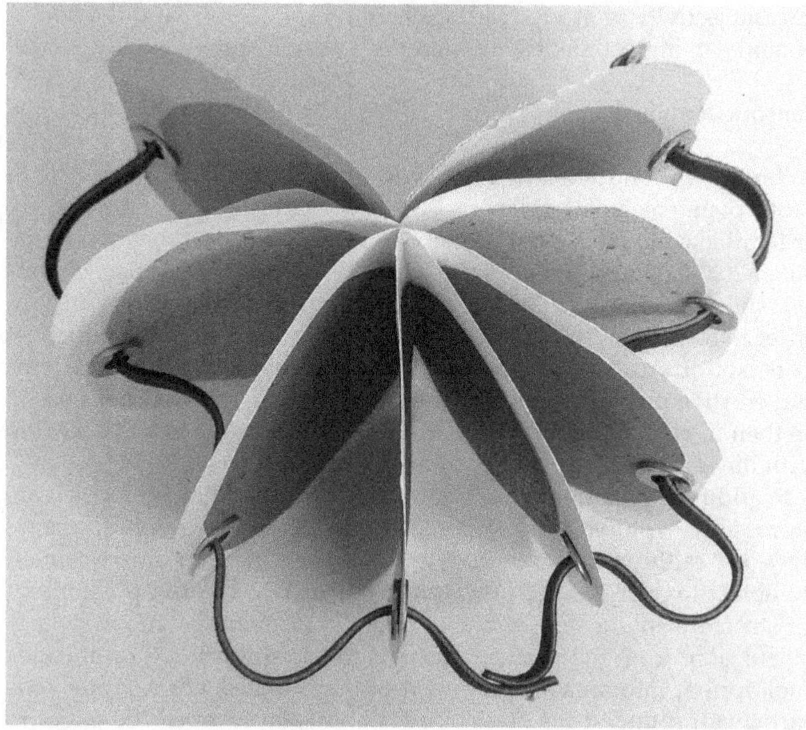

Figure 9.1: Anonymous workshop participant, *Untitled,* Paper, leather, and grommets, 6″ × 4″, 2021.

This is not to say that text was an unimportant aspect to the artists' books. Text features quite heavily in most of the participants' creations but in a less narrative format than typically seen in an autobiography. The freedom of freehand writing without a screen or ruled lines enabled the makers to use text more expressively: words are scattered around the page to reflect a bombardment of intrusive thoughts, particular words grow to engulf all other utterances, and sentences twist and meander across spreads. Like concrete poetry, the arrangement of text lends additional layers of meaning in excess to the literal definition of words (see Figure 9.2).

Although the placement of words may feel chaotic at times to reflect the disarray of that moment, working within a paginated form lent an inherent sense of organization to what may have remained stream-of-consciousness thoughts or pure emotion. Books require a certain amount of planning, and one of the most challenging aspects of creating these works was making decisions on how to distribute the visual and textual

Dendrites
The hospital is two hours away
STEEL PIN
COGNITIVE
BRAIN
I'll meet the stretcher vehicl
You can't live in a place with wood heat and no water
Axon
COGNITIVE IMPAIRMENT
I'll meet the stretcher
Axon
Terminal
I can't do this
STEEL PIN
Infection
Why were you on the roof

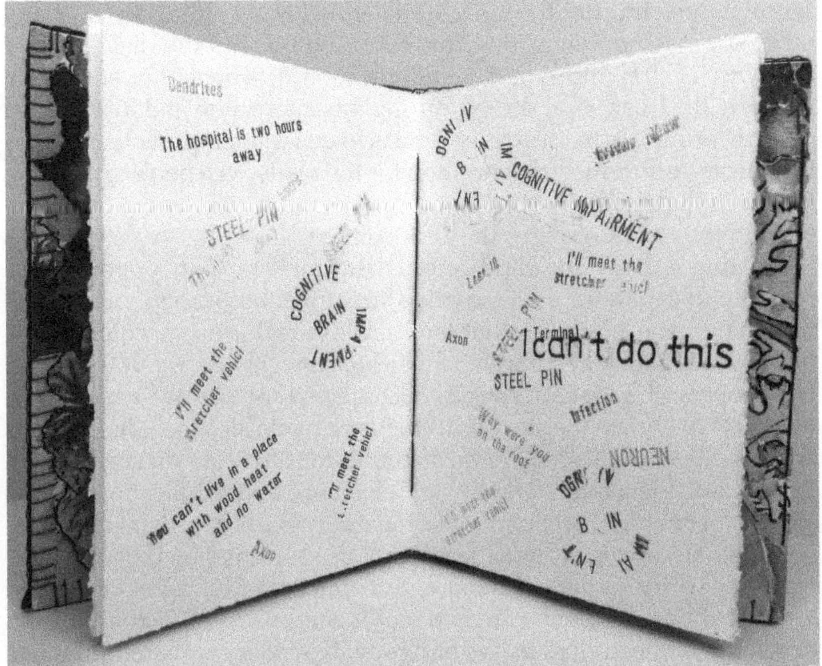

Figure 9.2: Leona M. Herzog, *Care Giving Care Giving Care*, Paper and ink, 8″ × 6″, 2022.

elements from beginning to end. The reflective process of organizing events, thoughts, or dialogue between the front and back covers of their books prompted a tacit order that ultimately aids in the comprehension of tumultuous circumstances – for both the makers and readers.

I challenged the participants to work within unconventional book structures like the do-si-do or French door formats, which both include two spines and two sets of pages within a single book entity. The goal of working with dualistic books was to promote multiple perspectives and ways of knowing. I prompted them to utilize this dualistic structure to portray, perhaps, what they said versus what they thought, a conversation between them and their healthcare provider, or a textual side and a sensory side. For example, one participant recounted a contentious conversation with her sceptical and dismissive neurologist. With her words on one set of pages and his words on the other, she attempts to convince the neurologist to do an additional MRI scan to prove that her hearing loss is linked to the progression of her multiple sclerosis. Reading both sets of pages one after the other, alternating between the halves, or any other approach to navigating this book complicates the dialogue and any sense of straightforward communication. The book thus effectively transfers the frustration she felt during this interaction and in the midst of her hearing loss to the reader, who is likewise attempting to decipher the narrative. Producing frustration for the reader in a book concerning frustration ultimately evokes a sense of empathy more holistically than reading the text as a single, linear document.

Creating a book by hand affords the makers with opportunities not only to capitalize on alternative structures but also to incorporate unconventional materials that evoke additional sensory communication. Particularly when participants were challenged to craft their own hard covers, they felted, sewed, decoupaged, or cut out ready-made materials to initiate the story within. Participants also included pockets and pouches to hold small loose materials for the reader to engage with throughout their read. These were elements that publication houses would not be able to accommodate. For example, one participant crafted her original X-ray films into the cover of her book and included various hand-sewn "tea pouches" filled with copper screws, coins, and dried lavender buds. These unconventional inclusions to a book are meant to conjure up healing practices and provide sensory care to the readers as they flip through the pages and waft in this relaxing, natural scent.

The final aspect of artists' books that is particular to the hand-crafted medium is the emphasis on performance. As the navigation of the book can be customized to suit the expression of the makers, their creations adopted elements of other kinds of print media like card games, take-aways, and puzzles. One participant used copious amounts of humour and a kind of gamification of her book to not only hold the reader's attention but also introduce a sense of play within the otherwise heavy topic of repeated concussions.

Pockets incorporated into the pages include felted interlocking pieces for you to solve the puzzle of her "fuzzy brain" while learning about the symptoms of concussions. Another pocket contains a concussion stamp card with progressive prizes like "Depression, headaches, balance issues, and much more! Ask *your* medical team for more information!" The use of humour and performance in this book invites the reader to engage with illness, rather than alienating the reader if the narrative becomes too much to handle (see Figure 9.3).

## Learning through Book-Bodies: Towards a Material Phenomenology

Instead of focusing on the text of these books, which also provides vivid and uncensored insights into what it is like to live with illness

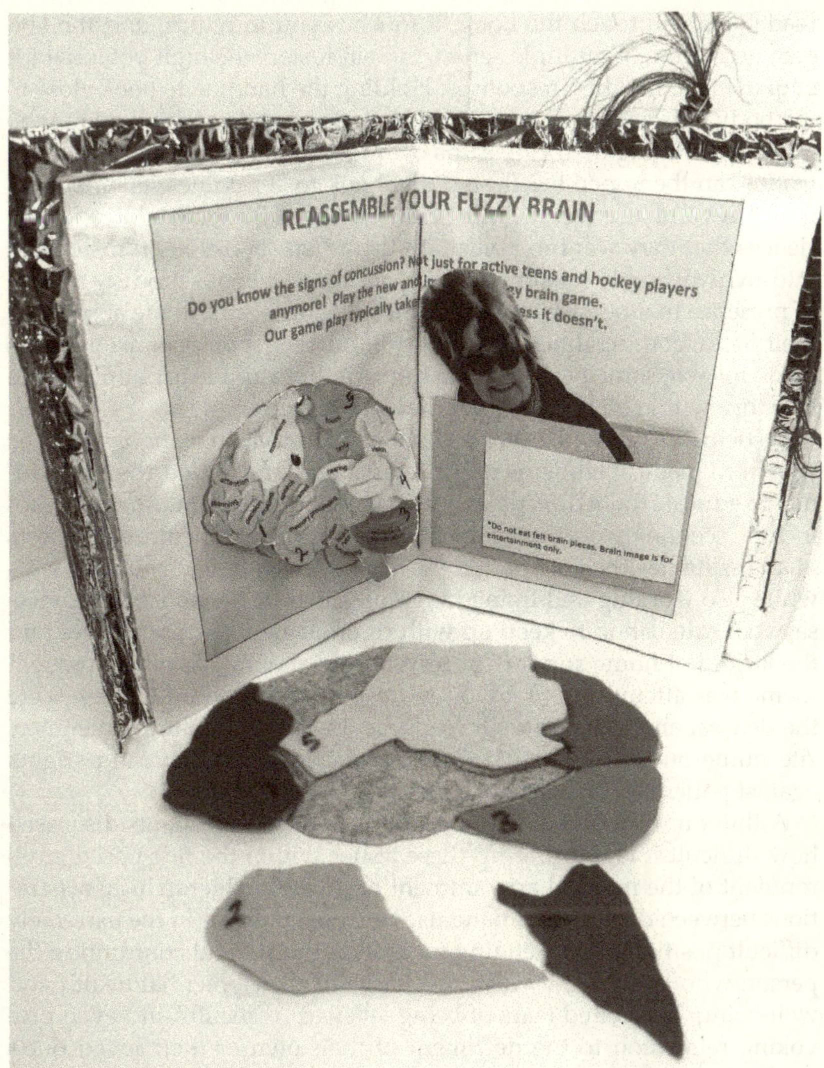


Figure 9.3: Anonymous, *Untitled*, Paper and multimedia, 8″ × 6″, 2022.

and disability, this chapter emphasizes the learning and intersubjective potential of handling multi-sensory book objects. Taking up the call of incorporating phenomenology as a powerful means of empathy-creation from physicians like Drew Leder and philosophers like Havi Carel, I argue that the artists' books these participants make actually foster a productive phenomenological connection between maker and reader. As you touch the book, it touches you in return, and the layered activation of multiple senses therein fosters the high potential for empathetic embodied responses. Holding the handmade book close to the body, it is as if you are slipping into the hands of the person who made it. Running their fingertips over the stitches along the spine, the reader can then open the flesh of the book to "examine" its innermost structures and discover the most vital aspects of the makers' lived experiences that they want to reveal. As the artists' books are transformed into archival bodily referents of their makers, the books produce a sense of presence that persists through time and space, and in the absence of their literal corporealities. The sense of touching a piece of art that was made for *you*, some person in the future to hold and learn from, makes the story within all the more visceral and urgent.

Participants took to heart the knowledge that their books will be shown to medical students and professionals and seized the opportunity to educate them directly about their experiences. Prominent themes include seemingly callous or uncaring physicians, difficulties and costs of accessing healthcare, or attempts to comply with medical treatments while also working and living in remote areas of Canada. Salient messages of exhaustion to keep up with rigorous treatment schedules and the lack of at-home support or respite care abound. Another frequent theme was attempting to advocate for a dying loved one. These were the densest and most difficult reads, as the surviving family members cite numerous examples of perceived racism, misogyny, and stigma against patients with substance use disorders.

Within our roundtable critiques of the books, participants discussed how difficult it is to bring up these issues within the fast-paced environment of the medical appointment or given the hierarchical separations between doctors and patients. This puts patients in the extremely difficult position of challenging medical authority and confronting the person who is, in many ways, in charge of their potential health and well-being. They cited fears of being labelled "difficult" and even provoking retaliation to the detriment of their own or their loved one's medical care. These slights have lingered in the participants' consciousness for years, even decades in some cases, and are felt afresh in the making of their books. If they could no longer tell the medical staff these things directly, then they were determined to tell the readers of their books, the next generation of physicians, what happened to them and their loved ones so these things might never occur again.

Being provided the opportunity and time to deeply consider the consequences of navigating the medical system within their artists' books fostered a sense of authority and power over situations in which the participants felt quite powerless. If the book is a material metaphor for the body, then taking control of the narrative and every other aspect of crafting their artist's book promoted a sense of bodily agency. I also assert that the form of the book as an icon of truth and publishable expertise in our culture also promotes a sense of authority to the expressions held within. The command the makers capture to express themselves within their books flips the hierarchies of knowledge between doctors and patients and prompts the reader to become a learner of others' lived experiences.

Although the *Embodied Books Archive* is still in its production phase and has yet to be fully integrated into medical humanities curricula, the potential for this collection is modelled on similar initiatives from the University of Kent's *Prescriptions Collection* in the United Kingdom and the University of New England's *Maine Women Writers Collection* (MWWC) in the United States. In particular, the MWWC's holdings of works by Martha Hall demonstrate the pedagogical value of archiving artists' books on the topics of illness within medical institutions. Although Hall died after her long illness with breast cancer in 2003, her books continue to speak to health sciences students and continuing education medical professionals every semester. The readers are prompted to spend intimate time with her books and listen to her poetic autobiographical experiences of illness and impending mortality before opening the room for group dialogue and private reflective response letters to the memory of Hall. The MWWC librarian Cathleen Miller and UNE professor Jennifer Tuttle who teach with these artist's books recount that "Hall's work provides students and practitioners with the important reminder of patients' subjectivity and of the dehumanizing experience of clinical encounters" (60), and that the readers "articulate their thanks for having found in her books a secure place to speak openly about mortality" (59).

While the permanence of books ensures the bookmaker's experiences may be called upon again and again, even decades beyond the physical body's ability to do so, I further assert that the diversity of voices and experiences available for learning also broadens from the inclusion of artists' books within library holdings. Aside from the multitude of barriers to formal publishing, the very act of writing a narrative, however short, may be an insurmountable hurdle for those whose stories are too intimate, too private, to be uttered. *Embodied Books* participants who wanted to express such difficult medical experiences in their artists' books found safe strategies to do so within the communicative potential of collage, drawing, materiality, and perhaps some guiding words. If this course centred written narrative as the de facto mode of expression, however poetic, I do not believe it would have been accessible to such participants, or they would have chosen a less vulnerable topic, and these valuable testaments of shame, tragedy, and resiliency would not be represented in the collection.

This is not to say that artists' books as a pedagogical medium do not include pitfalls. The most glaring critique of mobilizing this format in the medical humanities is that they require an in-person read to comprehend their full sensory meaning. As opposed to easily disseminated digital formats of narratives and literature, the physical form of artists' books severely limits the number of people who may be able to engage them. To overcome this hurdle, I provided enough materials for each participant to make two of each book: one to keep and share with loved ones and their health providers, and one to potentially donate to the *Embodied Books Archive*. Another format we utilized is a single-sheet folded zine, which is meant to be uploaded to our accessible website and printed off using a home printer in an unlimited edition. Finally, an online catalogue of the collection will include images of each book, with videos, readings, audio descriptions, and captions for each book in the works to make their digital presence as accessible and sensory as possible. This catalogue can be found at https://www.embodiedbooks.com.

Another critique of this medium for learning is that interpreting abstract artists' books in the absence of didactic language introduces a level of subjectivity that may be seen to take away from their pedagogical potential. After all, how can we know what it is like to live with, say, post-traumatic stress disorder, if the author doesn't exactly tell us? First, I respond that we can never truly know another person's experience, even with the most thorough description, because there is always going to be a kind of filtering and framing of these narratives through our own life experiences and imaginations. Second, I argue that because illness is an embodied experience, learning about its particularities in and through the body's senses is a powerful means of expression that does not have to rely on words. As described earlier, one participant's book does not simply recount a physician not listening to the patient's concerns of multiple-sclerosis-linked hearing loss but cuts the dialogue across two sets of pages too *evoke the sense of* miscommunication and frustration in the book's performance. It may surprise first-time artist's book readers just how much they can comprehend about another's experience using only the sensing body.

Finally, I argue that the potential pedagogical value of artists' books is not simply recounting a patient's experience but inviting each reader to add their own interpretation of the abstract book as a collective meaning-making process. Inserting one's own subjectivity between the pages of these books promotes a sense of dialogue with the maker, rather than a one-way transmission of knowledge. The reader becomes an active participant in the intersubjectivity of illness if they are tasked with making sense of the various artistic elements and putting forth an interpretation that may or may not align with the maker's intention. This process of hermeneutics was demonstrated within our roundtable critique procedure, in which a peer was charged with presenting another artist's book to the class and proposing a potential meaning for the work, and then opening the discussion of the book to the rest of the group. It was only after this group discussion that the author-maker was invited to provide any additional insight (if they wanted). This critique procedure has the dual benefit of retaining a sense of privacy for the maker if they do not want to talk directly about the inspiration behind the book and also showing how our own subjectivity produces multiple interpretations of illness experiences. In the end, none of the participants were upset if others didn't catch on to the intended meaning of their books. The delight of others accurately interpreting a book was equally matched by hearing a completely different take on the same set of pages. That being said, participants had the option to include very straightforward, explanatory narratives if they desired. The balance of abstraction and didactic expression was completely up to them and only added to the breadth of creative solutions for these works.

The procedure of materializing your own experiences through bookmaking and then witnessing others interpret your interpretation is a revelatory display of revealing biases and fostering empathy. I believe this intersubjectivity will have a profound effect on medical learners and address some of the most cited potential benefits of integrating humanities into medical curricula. Everyone in the room will flex their senses of discovery in the co-creation of meaning, sit with ambiguity, and acknowledge that multiple perspectives can be right and true at the same time. They will hear and feel experiences that are radically different from their own and gain exposure to some of the root causes of medical discontent like speed, discrimination, and lack of resources. Prompted by these artists' books, learners may initiate reflexive dialogues on what to do within their own roles as physicians if and when they encounter similar circumstances and cultivate humanistic competencies for patient engagement and support.

Within our group discussion and anonymous surveys, I asked the participants what they hoped would happen by donating their books to the collection, knowing they will be mobilized within medical humanities curricula. One participant notes that the books "could transform these negative healthcare experiences into positive activism." Another hopes to emphasize "that we are more than symptoms, disease and illness. That the experience we have with healthcare providers has long-term implications and may create barriers to wellness and to participation in treatment." By literally objectifying their experiences of medicine and illness into a book, they hope to spark dialogue on practising holistic care, perpetually remind physicians that patients are so much more than a diagnosis, and for them to become competent and compassionate physicians.

## Conclusion

Although illness narratives are already well integrated into medical humanities curricula, I aim for the *Embodied Books* project to provide a substantial rationale for including artists' books as another primary resource of learning about the patient experience. For one, bookmaking was found to be an approachable and accessible format to express medical experiences with creative agency and sensory allure. The vast majority of the nineteen participants did not consider themselves artists, nor had most been familiar with the medium of artists' books before deciding to sign up for the course. Nevertheless, the familiarity of books as objects of learning and their incorporation of intuitive communication strategies like image, touch, texture, sound, scent, time, and performance led the participants to customize their books with a range of expressive modalities that felt right for them. With so many artistic options for creating meaning, makers do not have to attain an academic level of writing or artistry to formulate the events of their life into a comprehensible book. Therefore, the breadth of illness expression may ultimately be much wider than narrative can capture alone.

Without the time constraints of a medical appointment or the social proprieties and pressures within the doctor-patient relationship, the makers were empowered to lay bare the real barriers and frustrations they face within the medical system. Likewise, the readers of these books will not be under pressure to "fix" or "solve" the problem at hand, but only to listen and imagine themselves in similar circumstances and how they would want to be treated. Spending time with patient-made artists' books, hearing and feeling their stories of medicine anew, and allowing oneself to feel the emotions they bring up is a potentially transformative practice of countering the depersonalizing effects of modern medicine for patient and practitioner alike. Such a reflexive engagement with artists' books has the potential to alert medical learners to disparities experienced by patients and, ultimately, apply more empathetic and accommodating care in their future practices. For the makers, the meditative time spent reflecting on their lives and crafting their book-bodies created space for creative flourishing and well-being in the midst of ailing health and for new and productive meanings of illness to take hold.

## WORKS CITED

Bolaki, Stella, and Egidija Ciricaite. *Prescriptions: Artists' Books on Wellbeing and Medicine*. Natrix Natrix Press, 2017.

Carel, Havi. *Phenomenology of Illness*. Oxford UP, 2016.

Leder, Drew. *The Distressed Body*. U of Chicago P, 2016.

Tuttle, Jennifer S., and Cathleen Miller. "Unruly Voices: Artists' Books and Humanities Archives in Health Professions Education." *Journal of Medical Humanities*, vol. 41, 2020, pp. 53–64, https://doi.org/10.1007/s10912-019-09599-1, Medline:31903517.

# 10 The Otherness of Fat: An Intersectional Psychotherapy Story

HILARY OFFMAN

"If you haven't had sex like this, then you haven't lived." Emily proceeded to describe in exquisite and graphic detail the best sex she'd ever had during a torrid affair with her new, hot, married lover and to delineate exactly why I couldn't relate to it because I clearly wasn't passionate enough. Feelings of shame, humiliation, and confusion rose up in me as she spoke.

Why was Emily saying this? Was she trying to make me feel inferior? At that moment, it certainly felt that way – I suddenly sensed I had landed in some kind of unannounced competition. And why was this coming up now? A few years before, Emily would never have said such a thing. I wondered what had changed and whether Emily was right about me. Was I simply not a passionate person?

Literary narratives can provide us with indispensable insight into how otherness impacts subjective experience. Narratives in the form of psychotherapy stories offer a unique opportunity to explore experiences of otherness via a therapist's intimate immersion in how being different directly impacts their patients. But until now, most psychotherapy stories have typically neglected any direct consideration of how discrepancies in power and privilege intersect to affect the therapeutic process and, by extrapolation, othered life in general. To facilitate an awareness of how otherness impacts patients, we need not only stories that consider how the shame and stigma associated with otherness create intersectional experience but also narratives that include the intimate self-awareness of the treating therapist. A psychotherapy story that incorporates details of a therapist's own participation in the creation of her patient's narrative (Aron 291; Hoffman 25–30) can help us grasp how otherness can come to define an entire life, situating both physician and patient in a sociocultural milieu that warrants deeper exploration.

Stigma can be said to exist when elements of labeling, stereotyping, status loss and discrimination occur together in a power situation that allows them (Link and Phelan 377). Stigma can be either hidden but "discreditable" if discovered, or readily visible and already "discredited" (Goffman 4). Regardless of the degree of visibility, it takes a societal power differential to stigmatize, construct stereotypes, and fully implement the disapproval, rejection, exclusion, and discrimination associated with stigma. When stigmatized individuals accept society's negative beliefs about themselves (Herek 910), interpersonal marginalization becomes intrapersonal, creating even more intense levels of shame and internalized stigma (Logie et al. 6). Furthermore, because our perceptions of stigmas are already imbued with value, the judgments we make about stigmatized individuals are often so automatic that we typically don't even notice, let alone question them (Alcoff 185).

Shame is often described as one of the most painful emotions a person can endure and includes feelings of unremitting despair, unworthiness, and a deep sense of unlovability (DeYoung 20). Shame and shaming are also inextricably linked with social inequality, frequently deployed to control and regulate those who exist outside of pervasive societal norms (Shefer and Munt 146). In addition, as shame has become increasingly dominant as the primary agent of social control in contemporary Western society, its articulation has become more taboo, making it even more likely to be rendered invisible (Scheff, "Goffman on Emotions" 116–17). In that sense, having feelings of shame for having feelings of shame further promotes keeping those feelings hidden from others (Kaufman 4). It's not surprising, then, that even in a psychotherapy context, both patients and therapists can go to great lengths to evade these distressing emotions.

The key to understanding the relationship between shame and stigma depends on the degree to which any given stigma is associated with responsibility and self-blame (Lewis 207). Thus, diminished identities that are perceived as someone's fault, such as body size, are associated with even greater levels of shame. It's not surprising, then, that shame is frequently at the very heart of enactments that occur when these marginalized identities come into play during psychotherapy.

In psychoanalysis and psychotherapy, an enactment can be thought of as an incident (misunderstanding, conflict, surprise) that occurs between a therapist and patient before either of them understands what is happening or why (Maroda 520). Since both patients and therapists have unconscious minds, the meaning of what transpires between them may not always be consciously accessible to either. While past iterations of enactments have tended to depict them as problems to be avoided at all costs – as if such a thing were remotely possible – in a contemporary psychoanalytic perspective, therapists are encouraged to make use of their subjectivity to unpack enactments' meanings. In that way, therapists can make productive use of enactments by exploring how patients might be thinking and feeling about them as therapists (known as transference) and how they, as therapists, might be thinking and feeling about their patients (known as countertransference).

Enactments are crucial to psychotherapy, because in the face of what patients may not yet understand or be able to articulate about themselves (unformulated experience) (Stern 1–2), enactments can represent the only access to pertinent, but still opaque, parts of patients' lives. Thus, even when enactments are disconcerting, they can still turn out to be exceedingly valuable by giving us access to unformulated experience that we can then examine intersubjectively by using the transference-countertransference matrix. However, when enactments involve feelings of shame that are mutually experienced by patients and therapists, they can be much harder to figure out.

That's because when patients and therapists share a diminished identity, the potential is created for that shame to be multiplied across their relationship, resulting in enactments that can threaten to derail almost any treatment. Under these circumstances, both therapists and patients can end up trying to circumvent any attempts to understand what "really" happened between them, unconsciously looking for workarounds that allow them to evade painful feelings of shame. At best, such avoidance can result in a lost opportunity to make use of the transference-countertransference matrix to understand something important. At worst, it can mean a volatile end to what might have otherwise been a highly productive therapeutic relationship.

The term *intersectionality* was coined by critical race theorist Kimberlé Crenshaw (1242) to describe how inequality and discrimination are determined by a complex interplay between socially-constructed identities. Intersectionality teaches us that "the organization of power [is] better understood as being shaped not by a single axis of social division ... but by many axes that work together and influence each other" (Collins and Bilge 2). In that sense, the diminished status associated with having more than one marginalized identity is not merely additive but greater than the sum of its parts (Collins and Bilge 8; Crenshaw 1244).

Societal norms create intersectional experience by maintaining the power of the status quo, whereby some of us are valued over and above others (Layton 239–40). We are all socialized to understand which identities are typically idealized and which are devalued (Frommer 34;

Layton 240). Even before entering school, children have internalized the "discrimination structure" of the society in which they are raised (Fors 109), and "normative unconscious processes" uphold these social norms, forming an automatic desire to belong to a favoured group (Layton 242). The immense privilege that accrues from conformity to these societal norms is often invisible to those who possess it, at least not until that privilege is questioned or put at risk. But whether we recognize them or not, the power differentials associated with these splits are always at hand, impacting us as we attempt to minimize the shameful narcissistic injury associated with objectionable otherness status.

When both patients and therapists are diminished by a marginalized intersectional identity, the potential is created for even more intense enactments. When therapists and patients share shame states, intersectional shame that resides in and is disavowed by both can cause an exponentially potent disruption. The more either exists in a state of continuous shame, the more each may generate shame in the other, producing a "triple spiral of shame within and between them, a state of individual and shared shame, which has no natural limit of intensity or duration" (Scheff, "Editor's Introduction" 1056). In this way, intersectional axes of difference that co-produce diminished social status within an individual can multiply interactively across individuals who share that same marginalized status.

Accounts of the psychological impact of embodied difference have tended to lack any input from those critically situated within that inequality (Watermeyer and Swartz 165). When Crenshaw explicitly situated herself as a Black woman within her own intersectional narrative, she indicated a "particular epistemological stance [that highlights the value of] experience and embodied knowledge" (Collins and Bilge 82). Intersectionality thus upholds the significance of individual experience by incorporating both the different experiences of "individual knowers" and an understanding of how these "knowers" are best positioned to challenge and create that knowledge.

Given that intersectionality privileges this proximity to lived experience, it offers a promising lens through which to examine power and privilege in the therapeutic relationship. A literary narrative with an intersectional lens can highlight how varying combinations of class, gender, race, sexuality, and body differentially position each individual, helping us understand how aspects of stigmatized otherness interact to confer diminished power and privilege via society's generalized assumptions about inherent inferiority (Livneh et al. 93; Smith 61).

When Emily informed me that I wasn't erotic or sensual enough to fully understand her, it made me think further about who and what my patients see when they come to me for psychotherapy. Many psychoanalysts show their respect for Freud by displaying curated volumes of his works, African artifacts, or Persian rugs. Identifying as a bit of an iconoclast, I prefer a playful, slightly disobedient interpretation. My mouse pad boasts a replica of Freud's carpet, a Freud bendy-figure proudly holds a pencil from its namesake's Vienna Museum, and an original 1963 movie poster entitled "Freud: The Secret Passion" adorns my wall. The poster is oversized, boldly colourful and scandalously suggestive, with gigantic beehive hairdos. The caption screams "He dared to search beyond the flesh!" My love for the poster's bold mid-century vibe has never extended to the lustful longing the poster promises, and depictions of a woman exerting that much effort to entice a man have never been my idea of hotness. Or so I thought.

As Emily's sexual exploits suggested, this was not the case for her. Emily had been referred to me many years before, having been diagnosed with numerous psychiatric problems including panic, bipolar, and borderline personality disorders. When I met her in her early 20s, Emily had already been married and divorced, had spent several months in a residential psychiatric treatment centre, and had moved back to her mother's place repeatedly, always on a moment's notice. She would engage in tumultuous or risky sexual relationships and then run away from the fallout. She found jobs, then quit them in volatile ways that usually involved telling her bosses "where to go." Eventually, Emily's life stabilized to such a degree that the idea that she had ever been diagnosed with borderline personality disorder seemed preposterous. In fact, it seemed that in many ways, Emily had become more and more like me, especially since I was fat, and Emily was gaining weight rapidly.

With our growing alikeness, Emily and I were convinced that she was getting better, despite our mutual weight problem. No longer emotionally or behaviourally volatile, she approached her life with a mature thoughtfulness that had me feeling like an exceedingly effective therapist. We felt closer in our relationship, and Emily often spoke about how if we had met under different circumstances, we would have become fast friends. And we needed each other: we seemed to be the only two "fat and fabulous" women amidst a sea of slim, fit, downtown professionals, and only we two could truly understand what this meant. But despite our areas of success, neither of us could seem to lose weight, and we both sensed our physical selves were starting to get out of control. At times our relationship felt almost like a secret romance, one that we both believed would never end. But like all romances, our relationship was destined for some tumultuous times.

When the Canadian government began to fund the costs of weight loss surgery, I began to consider it as a potentially viable option. I felt compelled to share this information with Emily, especially since she had already considered paying privately to have the surgery outside the country. When Emily found out that I was involved in the assessment process, she set the ball rolling to get her surgery as soon as possible. In contrast to Emily, and in keeping with my more cautious personality and growing apprehension, I began to slow down my own pursuit of surgery, terrified not only about potentially dangerous complications but also about the potentially devastating loss of the enjoyment of eating. For the first time in our relationship, Emily openly displayed her transferential frustration with me as she demanded to know when I would finally find the courage to make my decision about the surgery. She made it very clear that she was not impressed with my ambivalence and that the bloom was finally off the rose of our idealized romance.

Emily had her gastric bypass, while I dropped out of the program altogether. She sailed through surgery and lost weight rapidly (despite defiantly trying to eat a burger less than two weeks afterwards). Emily seemed to disappear in front of my very eyes, but as I witnessed her transformation, I found myself feeling sad to lose my connection to the twin she no longer was. She now seemed so far removed from my own choices that it felt as if I was looking at her through the wrong end of binoculars. In time, a gorgeous male colleague at her workplace expressed his overwhelming desire for her by physically lifting her up and holding her against the wall. Emily experienced an intense rush, feeling physically and emotionally lighter than she had ever been. No man, including her father, had ever picked her up with such delight. From that moment on, she was entirely hooked, and a torrid affair developed.

I observed and listened with dismay as Emily appeared to revert into the person I had first met years before, and more and more unlike the woman she had become under my charge. Her affair took centre stage during our sessions. In order to feel even more attractive, Emily underwent extensive and painful plastic surgery that she could not afford and spent much time focusing on her clothes and appearance. I witnessed her dresses become shorter and her cleavage deeper. Emily frequently demanded that I condone her affair, frustrated that I refused to collude with her pervasive lying and betrayal of her husband. She insinuated (correctly) that I was envious of her new body and the constant attention she encouraged and received from men, though I refused to confirm these transferential suspicions. Instead, I often found myself overwhelmed with countertransferential feelings of losing in a competition that I couldn't even believe I had entered. But because my feelings of shame were too painful, at this point, I was completely unable to reflect on why.

While in the past I had looked forward to sessions with Emily, I was ashamed to realize that I had come to dread them, especially since they were now filled with discussions of how convinced she was that she was having much better sex than I was. Emily had once been someone who shared my experience of inhabiting a diminished position in the eyes of the world. But now that she had the option, it felt like she was all too willing to abandon me for the preferred ranks of the normative, relishing the opportunity to feel better about herself specifically in comparison to me. My countertransference feelings of betrayal had me resenting her more and more intensely. Having triumphed over me, her transferential feelings of contempt had her feeling fed up.

During this period, Emily received a disturbing phone call from her mother. Sensing that her mother was saying her goodbyes, Emily immediately rushed to her side. Because of her deteriorating health, Emily's mother had been unable to travel for some time, so this meeting represented the first and only occasion she witnessed the astounding transformation of her daughter's physicality. Emily had dreamed of proving to her mother that she would prevail in her epic battle with her weight, but this sense of triumph lasted only a few hours. It turned out that Emily's mother had already decided that rather than waiting for her disease to claim her, she would take her own life. When Emily and her sister learned of the plan, they insisted she not do it alone. Their mother's response was, "Well, since you're both here, how about tonight?"

Emily's mother did die that night, but not without unforeseen complications. The three women held a farewell party, complete with a last meal and their mother's favourite candy for dessert. Pills that had been hoarded for months were ostensibly taken by the mother's own hand, even though that very hand had not been able to move on its own for a long time. Stories were told with laughter and tears. In the wee hours, Emily and her sister watched as their mother's breathing became progressively shallower, but as dawn threatened to bring with it caregivers – who would surely call the paramedics – Emily and her sister began to panic. According to Emily, her sister took it upon herself to hasten death in ways that even now, neither has ever spoken about, and the following day was filled with investigations by the coroner and police. It was fortunate that few questions were asked, and no charges were brought against them.

When Emily disclosed to her husband what had transpired, he was enraged that she had put herself and their family in jeopardy without discussing it with him first. Though not morally opposed to her mother's decision, I reacted in much the same way, alarmed to contemplate the narrowly missed criminal ramifications. I was furious that Emily's mother had allowed her children to participate in such a risky action without considering the potential danger to them and was appalled that Emily had taken part with so little thought. Emily felt utterly betrayed by both her husband and me.

With the threat of her mother's disapproval no longer looming, Emily's affair took on a new level of intensity and risk such that the discrepancy between our lifestyles enlarged further. When I finally did summon the courage to face the physical and emotional risks of my own surgery, I assumed it wouldn't be long until our bodies looked similar again. But fate dictated that because of my past surgical history, I had a different procedure than Emily's, continuing our separate trajectories. Although I lost some weight, it was not even close to the amount or the speed of Emily's weight reduction. Meanwhile, now that binge eating was no longer an option for Emily, binge drinking seemed to take over. Instead of recapturing our alikeness as I anticipated, Emily and I were continuing to cultivate difference, and I found myself worrying – maybe even hoping – that the excitement and freedom of her new life would catch up with her. On the two-year anniversary of her mother's death, my concerns were vindicated.

On that fateful night, Emily's lover cancelled plans with her at the last minute, and she was incensed by this reneging on his promise. She started drinking and driving from one friend's house to another, taking refuge with one, making sexual advances on another. Eventually, with an alcohol level double the legal limit, Emily drove straight into a tree. No one was injured but the car was totalled, and Emily was arrested and charged with impaired driving.

The next morning, things went from bad to worse. I received an urgent phone call from Emily's husband and when I returned it, I heard only sobbing and pleading through the line. Though I initially assumed her husband had found out about the affair, I learned instead that Emily had taken an overdose of prescription medication and was in the process of being rushed to hospital. Emily had never engaged in this kind of self-harm before, and I was scared. I cancelled my patients and drove across the city to the hospital, not knowing what I would find or what I could do.

In an emergency room bed, without her makeup or fashionable clothes, Emily appeared very young and very small. Despite the overdose, it became apparent that Emily had not intended to take her own life. Instead, she was evading the mortifying shame she had felt when she awoke the morning after her arrest. My heart broke as I began to think about the ways in which our mutual distancing, embedded in a transference-countertransference enactment so challenging that we couldn't yet approach it, might have contributed to this painful moment. I wondered how we could have come so far, only to seemingly end up back where we started? And perhaps an even more critical question – how did our mutually unconscious expression of these feelings develop into such an explosive enactment? Emily was deeply touched that I had dropped everything to be with her on that dreadful day, and we began the slow process of reflecting on what had transpired between us.

Before Emily lost weight, it seemed clear to me that I had helped her to self-actualize as I basked in the countertransferential glow of her increasing identification with me. Personally, I had always longed for someone who would truly understand what it felt like to be like me, "successful but fat" – earnestly admired for my visible accomplishments but judged for my visible failings. Such "trauma-generated longings for twinship" often give rise to dissociative processes that make it hard to see and accept differences (Brothers 393). Having someone like Emily idealize me by choosing my choices was a soothing antidote to the shame I felt for being visibly flawed and alleviated some of my anger at being judged as not good enough.

But after her massive weight loss, the shame that resided in me for being a failure was no longer attenuated by our similarity. As the sole remaining qualifier for intersectional status as a fat woman (Prohaska and Gailey 5; Van Amsterdam 155), I felt abandoned and alone. I also felt countertransferential disgrace for being the kind of analyst who envied my patient so much that I couldn't be sure whether I wanted Emily to get better or worse. When a therapist realizes that her ability to fulfill her clinical role depends on getting something so fundamental from her patient, the shame can be too overwhelming to acknowledge, even privately (Morrison 70).

As our differences emerged, we started to poke more provocatively at one another. One of the things Emily missed most about her relationship with her mother was their ability to have "knockdown, drag-out" fights that gloriously confirmed that nothing she could do or say would rupture their strong attachment. My developmental experience was of a mother who ardently refused to fight with me, insisting it was because I never made her angry! In my family, generations of women had swallowed their anger for the greater good, so it made sense how uncomfortable my growing resentment of Emily made me feel. When Emily commented how I never seemed to turn on the heat in my office, I accused her of rubbing it in that her slim body was no longer perpetually overheated. The presence of intense feelings of countertransference envy that I couldn't hide left me feeling increasingly humiliated in Emily's presence.

The intensity of our shared shame experience compelled me to face the harsh reality that Emily's drastic and breakneck weight loss had been harder for me, as evidenced by our transference-countertransference-based enactment, than I could admit to her or even to myself. My own change was characteristically slow – it took me several years to achieve the degree of weight loss that Emily had stampeded through. Meanwhile, like most Roux-en-Y gastric bypass patients, and because of her increasing alcohol consumption, Emily started to gain weight back, and over time the gap between us narrowed. As our weights became comparable, I found myself acting more boldly and with less restraint, becoming more interested in how I dressed and what I wore, now imitating Emily.

Meanwhile, completely out of the blue, one of my favourite psychoanalytic authors saw something in me that rekindled passions I did not know I had lost. This had nothing to do with my sexuality or my changing body image but with his regard for my mind and my writing. In high school, I had begun to develop a writing style that employed psychodynamic connections, something highly unusual for someone my age. But since I wanted, above all, to go to medical school, I failed to grasp how my decision to exchange creative development for the higher grades needed for admission might impact me overall. When this author took the initiative to read my first (and what I assumed would be my last) published psychoanalytic paper, I was amazed. When he told me how much he loved it, I was astounded. This recognition unleashed surprisingly powerful feelings in me, retrospectively reawakening a dormant desire to claim my own passionate voice. It also offered me a glimpse into how Emily might have felt the day her lover picked her up and held her so passionately against the wall. For the first time, I understood how Emily "fell," and I had to concede that I, too, could have surrendered to such a feeling. I couldn't help but recall my denial of the erotic appeal of the poster in my office, "Freud: The Secret Passion," nor obscure any longer the existence of a secret self who had related to it all along. Now the essential question for me was whether to confess this realization to Emily in the service of working out what had happened. I felt a personal need to come clean with her as a way of correcting the power differential derived from pretending that I was better than she was.

Emily soon noticed that something was up with me – she claimed that I seemed different to her, and she wanted to know why. In the spirit of unpacking our intense transference-countertransference-based enactment, I decided to tell her how I had changed my mind about how she had responded to her lover's overtures, admitting that my judgment of her was more to do with my own envy and feelings of abandonment than any actual moral superiority. We talked about how, on an unconscious level, I had convinced myself that her "out of control" behaviour had nothing to do with me, and that I had been merely an innocent bystander.

I also did my best to self-reflect on how aspects of my personal story might have contributed to dissociating from Emily's feelings and how our historical similarities might have contributed to our process (Maroda 520). Like Emily, I had also struggled for fatherly recognition but eventually concluded that my father had no interest in confirming anyone's subjectivity but his own. Though my unique talents for mirroring and validating often proved advantageous to him, they still felt insufficient to render my subjectivity worthy of adequate recognition. In contrast, I inferred that attention or interest of any kind would always be reserved for my mother, the perpetually perfect objectified woman with whom my "subjectified" self knew I could never compete.

Since I assumed I wasn't a good-enough object of desire for my father any more than Emily was for hers, it never occurred to me that my mother might have actually considered me a "worthy opponent." Now that I am at least as slim as Emily and can, therefore, allow myself to feel and display my desire without fear of inevitable humiliation, I can appreciate why my mother felt unsettled by how much my father and I were alike in humour and temperament, and how easily I could entice him into mischief in ways she never could. But back then, when she efficiently shut down my "alluring" behaviour with her formidable, sanctioning glance, I automatically took her disapproval as evidence that my aroused and unrestrained self required urgent renunciation. I never questioned my conviction that good women and good mothers should long for nothing but their children's success and happiness. As far as I was aware, the privilege of other appetites belonged only to boys. All I could consciously want was for my mother to think I was a "good girl," just like her.

Just like Emily's mother, mine also concealed her even occasional longings to attend to her own needs and wishes over mine. How relieved I would have been to have learned that I wasn't the only "wantonly" desirous female in town, rather than deeming myself a reject who couldn't even get her father to want her. The cumulative experience of feeling like an "oedipal loser," one who never experiences the sexual power and potency of even an occasional oedipal victory, can leave a girl feeling entirely without the power to "attract, entice and allure" (Davies 10). For little girls like Emily and me, the experience of not being enough to command fatherly recognition laid down the perfect foundation for further shame and humiliation. Emily's lover, and their heated sex life, permitted her to dissociate from the pain of having been abandoned by her tragic mother and to identify finally with her triumphant father. Seeing herself as capable of redeeming this victory out of the ashes of feeling like a loser represented a powerful corrective to what had been an unbearable sense of otherness. But in our complex transference-countertransference matrix, Emily's triumph simultaneously highlighted my own unbearable sense of failure. It made sense, then, that it took something radical to force me to face those excruciating feelings head on.

As a young girl, I had already developed atypical ideas about intimate relationships. When my friends proclaimed their absolute adoration for the pop heartthrob of the moment, I remember feeling confused, demanding to know why they liked him, though they had never even met. Similarly, I could not understand how a boy could fall in love from afar with a girl who did not even know he existed. To me, it seemed unfathomable to want someone based solely on their perceived value as an object rather than on a lived experience of that person. There was simply no way I was going to objectify any boy if he wasn't willing to "subjectify" *me* first, a sentiment to which I have remained true to this day. When I felt Emily was retaliating for how I had let her down, undoing all the mutual validation we had so carefully crafted together, at last, I was forced to fully confront difference in our relationship. I learned that Emily didn't at all share my insistence on being "subjectified" in intimate sexual relationships – nonetheless, as she regaled me with her heroic sexual activities, I felt belittled by her reminders that, unlike me, she was finally worthy of being objectified by a man.

Fat women are often characterized as failed women for simply not being good enough at being objects of desire. And if just being a fat woman isn't enough of a social disability (Herndon 123), being a fat woman who openly lusts is worse, since she is supposed to have relinquished her subjective longing as a consequence of her label, and by not complying, opens herself up to further ridicule and humiliation. Only women who possess wanted bodies are authorized to see themselves as "sexually entitled, to have desire and to display it openly" (Orbach 212). Because having, showing, and wanting to be the object of desire are all prohibited for fat women, it is understandable that a preoccupation with food can ironically end up serving as a sanctuary for appetites deemed unacceptable (Atlas 220). Unlike people, food never shames the eater for wanting it.

Shame creates the desire to disappear, to conceal oneself (Morrison 68) and now that Emily was no longer visibly fat, she took advantage of the opportunity to pretend she had never possessed this "discredited" identity (Goffman 4). In response, I rationalized that as the "boring, asexual" one with excellent insight, I was superior to her, the exciting, erotic one with poor judgment. To counter my profound shame for envying Emily, I needed to re-establish a sense of my *own* power – I needed to "win".

I could understand Emily's wish for a taste of the privilege we both craved, a chance to ally herself with the normative position given the opportunity for acquiring that "power by proxy" (Fors 105–7). But unlike those women who are ignorant of their "thin privilege" and therefore oblivious to their complicity in the oppression of fat women (Nash and Warin 76), Emily knew very well what it felt like to be on the receiving end of that kind of subjugation – thus, her triumph served to simultaneously highlight my own unbearable sense of failure. Given that we had shared marginalized intersectional status, it became impossible not to experience her abandonment of me as purposefully sadistic.

Emily fractured her ankle and came to a session just out of a cast, following several frustrating weeks of constrained freedom. Though she had emphatically denied that her injury related to alcohol misuse, privately I didn't believe her, though I didn't communicate this assumption. But spontaneously, and in a way that diverted from all I had been taught about "proper" psychoanalytic technique, I decided to ask her if it was really true – even though, or perhaps precisely because, doing so scared me. While I was now capable of "hiding" as much as Emily, I realized that I was not at all interested in taking advantage of that "privilege." With an anger I had previously heard about but never witnessed, Emily lashed out that she couldn't "fucking remember" how she fractured her ankle because she was "too fucking wasted," making clear that I had earned her wrath by posing the question in the first place. I agreed that my inquiry was intentionally provocative and admitted further that I was tired of pretending she was fooling me just to avoid conflict between us. I told her that what surprised me, however, was the relief rather than the upset I felt hearing her aggressive answer, and how much more authentic our relationship seemed when I admitted I wasn't interested in buying the "fabulous" self she was trying to sell me. I was modelling for Emily what it could look like to refuse to give up one's subjectivity without needing to retaliate against the one trying to shut it down. Later that day, instead of drinking away her feelings at a bar, Emily chose to go home and tell her family she needed to be alone to "eat bad pizza in [her] pajamas." She later described her awareness that she wanted to "stay mad" as a "strange turning point."

Within a few weeks, Emily found herself at yet another turning point. This time it was her adolescent son who was injured – but rather than staying home with him, she allowed herself to be lured by the bar. When his condition worsened and he was unable to contact her, she arrived home obviously drunk to find that he and his father had visited the hospital emergency room without her. Emily could not accept this parenting failure and, with my encouragement and support, agreed to go to her first Alcoholics Anonymous (AA) meeting. A couple of relapses later, I returned from vacation amazed to find her still engaged with AA and eager to talk about how it felt to spend time with "real people who were willing to put their shit on the fucking table." Although I liked what Emily was reporting, I reminded myself to remain sceptical and not succumb to the wishful thinking she so skilfully projected when she told me – and everyone else in her life – exactly what we wanted to hear. However, with mounting optimism and a spreading smile I noticed the ways in which this instance felt entirely different.

Now the Emily in front of me didn't seem to care whether she looked fabulous or not or that she hadn't conveyed the remotest interest in my trip as she typically would have. In fact, it was the first time she expressed the details of her own experience without letting me get a single word in edgewise, like an excited child making the luxurious assumption that her parent would enjoy every minute. I silently acknowledged the ironic pleasure of being objectified by someone who had always insisted on "subjectifying" me first, an experience I would previously never have dreamed of enjoying.

The literary narrative of a psychotherapy story can illustrate how the othered identities of both physician and patient may entwine and interact in complex ways that inevitably impact patient care. An intersectional lens highlights how the shame associated with marginalized identities is always part and parcel of the society in which we live. No one can escape the reality of the sociocultural discrepancies in power and privilege associated with the stigma of otherness.

Like our patients, therapists also have unconscious minds that do their best to avoid experiencing overwhelming feelings of shame. And when those feelings of shame are based on mutual intersectional experiences of otherness, they can be too intense to allow the unpacking of transference-countertransference reactions underlying a challenging enactment – that is, until something happens to dislodge us from such impasses. The reality is that though we may have been taught otherwise, it's crucial for therapists to acknowledge that we are no more able to stand outside our own histories and experiences than anyone else.

The good news is that we need not despair about this realization – we can choose to make use of it by worrying less about *whether* our subjectivity impacts our patients and more about *how* our personal history and experiences help us better comprehend theirs. Psychotherapy narratives that introduce us to the ways in which a physician's subjectivity might interact with that of their patient can provide us with precisely the kind of indispensable perspective that therapists have been trained to overlook. A health humanities perspective can help us re-conceptualize our challenging personal responses to our patients as an opportunity to become more attuned healthcare providers.

## WORKS CITED

Alcoff, Linda Martín. *Visible Identities: Race, Gender, and the Self.* Oxford UP, 2005.

Aron, Lewis. "The Patient's Experience of the Analyst's Subjectivity." *Psychoanalytic Dialogues*, vol. 1, no. 1, Jan. 1991, pp. 29–51. https://doi.org/10.1080/10481889109538884.

Atlas, Galit. "Sex and the Kitchen: Thoughts on Culture and Forbidden Desire." *Psychoanalytic Perspectives*, vol. 9, no. 2, Sept. 2012, pp. 220–32, https://doi.org/10.1080/1551806X.2012.716302.

Brothers, Doris. "Trauma, Gender, and the Dark Side of Twinship." *International Journal of Psychoanalytic Self Psychology*, vol. 7, no. 3, July 2012, pp. 391–405. https://doi.org/10.1080/15551024.2012.686155.

Collins, Patricia Hill, and Sirma Bilge. *Intersectionality.* John Wiley & Sons, 2020.

Crenshaw, Kimberle. "Mapping the Margins: Intersectionality, Identity Politics, and Violence against Women of Color." *Stanford Law Review*, vol. 43, no. 6, 1991, pp. 1241–99, https://doi.org/10.2307/1229039.

Davies, Jody Messler. "Falling in Love with Love Oedipal and Postoedipal Manifestations of Idealization, Mourning, and Erotic Masochism." *Psychoanalytic Dialogues*, vol. 13, no. 1, Feb. 2003, pp. 1–27, https://doi.org/10.1080/10481881309348718.

DeYoung, Patricia A. *Understanding and Treating Chronic Shame: A Relational /Neurobiological Approach*. Routledge, 2015.

Fors, Malin. *A Grammar of Power in Psychotherapy: Exploring the Dynamics of Privilege*. American Psychological Association, 2018.

Frommer, Martin Stephen. "Desire, The Social Unconscious, and Shame." *Psychoanalysis, Culture & Society*, vol. 12, no. 1, Apr. 2007, pp. 32–37, https://doi.org/10.1057/palgrave.pcs.2100106.

Goffman, Erving. *Stigma: Notes on the Management of Spoiled Identity.* Simon and Schuster, 1963.

Herek, Gregory M. "Confronting Sexual Stigma and Prejudice: Theory and Practice." *Journal of Social Issues*, vol. 63, no. 4, Dec. 2007, pp. 905–25, https://doi.org/10.1111/j.1540-4560.2007.00544.x.

Herndon, April. "Disparate but Disabled: Fat Embodiment and Disability Studies." *Nwsa Journal*, 2002, pp. 120–37.

Hoffman, Irwin Z. *Ritual and Spontaneity in the Psychoanalytic Process: A Dialectical-Constructivist View*. Routledge, 1998. https://doi.org/10.4324/9781315803371.

Kaufman, Gershen. *The Psychology of Shame: Theory and Treatment of Shame-Based Syndromes*. Springer Publishing Company, 2004.

Layton, Lynne. "Racial Identities, Racial Enactments, and Normative Unconscious Processes." *The Psychoanalytic Quarterly*, vol. 75, no. 1, Jan. 2006, pp. 237–69, https://doi.org/10.1002/j.2167-4086.2006.tb00039.x.

Lewis, Michael. *Shame: The Exposed Self*. Simon and Schuster, 1995.

Link, Bruce G., and Jo C. Phelan. "Conceptualizing Stigma." *Annual Review of Sociology*, vol. 27, no. 1, Aug. 2001, pp. 363–85, https://doi.org/10.1146/annurev.soc.27.1.363.

Livneh, Hanoch, et al. "Stigma Related to Physical and Sensory Disabilities." *The Stigma of Disease and Disability: Understanding Causes and Overcoming Injustices*, American Psychological Association, 2014, pp. 93–120, https://doi.org/10.1037/14297-006.

Logie, Carmen H., et al. "HIV, Gender, Race, Sexual Orientation, and Sex Work: A Qualitative Study of Intersectional Stigma Experienced by HIV-Positive Women in Ontario, Canada." *PLoS Medicine*, vol. 8, no. 11, 2011, p. 1–12. https://doi.org/10.1371/journal.pmed.1001124. Medline:22131907

Maroda, Karen J. "Enactment: When the Patient's and Analyst's Pasts Converge." *Psychoanalytic Psychology*, vol. 15, no. 4, 1998, p. 517, https://doi.org/10.1037/0736-9735.15.4.517.

Morrison, Andrew P. "The Analyst's Shame." *Contemporary Psychoanalysis*, vol. 44, no. 1, Jan. 2008, pp. 65–82, https://doi.org/10.1080/07351690.2024.2332148.

Nash, Meredith, and Megan Warin. "Squeezed between Identity Politics and Intersectionality: A Critique of 'Thin Privilege' in Fat Studies." *Feminist Theory*, vol. 18, no. 1, Apr. 2017, pp. 69–87. https://doi.org/10.1177/1464700116666253.

Orbach, Susie. "Coming into Desire." *Psychoanalytic Perspectives*, vol. 9, no. 2, Sept. 2012, pp. 209–14, https://doi.org/10.1080/1551806X.2012.716289.

Prohaska, Ariane, and Jeannine A. Gailey. "Theorizing Fat Oppression: Intersectional Approaches and Methodological Innovations." *Fat Oppression around the World*, Routledge, 2021, pp. 1–8.

Scheff, Thomas. "Goffman on Emotions: The Pride-Shame System." *Symbolic Interaction*, vol. 37, no. 1, Feb. 2014, pp. 108–21, https://doi.org/10.1002/symb.86.

Scheff, Thomas J. "Editor's Introduction: Shame and Related Emotions: An Overview." *American Behavioral Scientist*, vol. 38, no. 8, Aug. 1995, pp. 1053–59, https://doi.org/10.1177/0002764295038008002.

Shefer, Tamara, and Sally R. Munt. "A Feminist Politics of Shame: Shame and Its Contested Possibilities." *Feminism & Psychology*, vol. 29, no. 2, May 2019, pp. 145–56, https://doi.org/10.1177/0959353519839755.

Smith, Christine A. "Intersectionality and Sizeism: Implications for Mental Health Practitioners." *Women & Therapy*, vol. 42, no. 1–2, Apr. 2019, pp. 59–78. https://doi.org/10.1080/02703149.2018.1524076.

Stern, Donnel B. *Partners in Thought: Working with Unformulated Experience, Dissociation, and Enactment*. Routledge, 2010.

Van Amsterdam, Noortje. "Big Fat Inequalities, Thin Privilege: An Intersectional Perspective on 'Body Size.'" *European Journal of Women's Studies*, vol. 20, no. 2, May 2013, pp. 155–69, https://doi.org/10.1177/1350506812456461.

Watermeyer, Brian, and Leslie Swartz. "Disablism, Identity and Self: Discrimination as a Traumatic Assault on Subjectivity." *Journal of Community & Applied Social Psychology*, vol. 26, no. 3, May 2016, pp. 268–76. https://doi.org/10.1002/casp.2266.

# Afterword

EFTIHIA MIHELAKIS AND LUCILLE TOTH

Superiority? Inferiority?

Why not simply try to touch the other, feel the other, discover each other?

Was my freedom not given me to build the world of you ... ?

At the end of this book we would like the reader to feel with us the open dimension of every consciousness.

– Fanon, *Black Skin, White Masks*

Health and illness alter the ways in which our bodies (including our brains) accommodate and create meaning. Interestingly – and far from what common sense would purport – it is the very ambiguity of meaning that is empathy building. Following Fanon's ambition to use the act of creating/writing as a form of narrative repair for both marginalized individuals and communities at large, our book openly and critically engages with textual expressions of health and illness. These expressions can be approached as perceptual encounters allowing readers an opportunity to feel the complex dimensions of our bodies and our subjectivities. Encountering these narratives is a chance to share moments with those with whom we may not be meant to collide, with times and spaces we might not otherwise experience. It is these different dimensions of consciousness (to quote Fanon again) where proximity between other cultural and linguistic worlds with otherworldly states of mind, of being, of (barely) existing, can come together. Literary texts unfold dimensions of consciousness as "perceptual dimensions" (Gagnon Chainey), whether they unravel the aesthetic dimensions of the bodily experience of syphilis, cancer, HIV/AIDS, hygiene, mental health, diabetes, and so much more, literary texts expand embodied experiences of health and illness. In short, literary studies is a physical practice that cannot exist without the closeness of health and illness.

Our aspiration with this book was to broaden and explore new avenues for literary studies while contemplating the potential for transnational perspectives on embodied narratives. Each chapter of *Embodied Narratives in the Health Humanities and Literary Studies* has offered bold perspectives on how embodiment generates narratives of health, contributing to a diverse collection of transdisciplinary scholarship spanning the intersections of cognitive neuroscience and fiction, from the nuanced portrayal of historical figures, the exploration of Japanese American experiences post-World War II, the medical and social complexities of the COVID-19 pandemic, the multifaceted dimensions of graffiti activism in Senegal, the democratization of healthcare through DIYAPS, the transformative potential of artists' books in medical education, to the intricate dynamics of psychotherapeutic interactions. Collectively, these chapters underscore the importance of transdisciplinary scholarship in which literary studies are interwoven with the health humanities. These artist-writer-scholars have addressed social, cultural, and health issues and opened up bold avenues for understanding the (not so) human experience of health. Adopting a health humanities perspective allows us to embrace the inherent complexities of therapeutic interactions and enrich the therapeutic process, enabling healthcare providers to become more sensitive and responsive practitioners. In essence, these chapters emphasize the transformative power of literary texts in shaping our understanding of ourselves, our communities, and the world around us. Whether through fiction, historical narratives, activism, or therapeutic journeys, literary studies serve as a powerful tool for fostering empathy, challenging societal norms, and empowering individuals to enact change.

The authors in this book have tried to direct attention to relations with bodily experiences by opening up the ways that translingual and transnational literary texts interlock affective dimensions of public health with historically precarious, marginalized voices and bodies who have been and still are misnamed or unnamed or whose name/ing remains in the discretion of the attending physician, promote insight, action, and unrest. Paying attention to these ways of noticing with a language that is literary in nature will not as readily efface the hegemonic structure of health institutions, nor will it serve as a remedy to social and economic inequities. While such noticing can represent an alternative, or even a subversive form of perceiving alterity, it should not be taxed with the responsibility of solving these issues. In this way, this book exemplifies a relation to literature that may not be relevant for use in a world where its cultural capital has been judged insufficient in the media and in the academe. To know that the body is perceived through our word-filled relations to health and illness and actualized through our reading and writing of the body is to acknowledge that we are looking for "true moral complexity" and this is "rarely found in simple reversals" (Nelson 13) of fate or conditions. These readings open us to something that is opaque, unhinged, and unfinished.

Our hope is that this book opens perceptual dimensions between empathy and proximity, phenomenology and materiality, language and cruelty; that it can teach us to live in a sustained vulnerability that health and illness narratives address but that society often negates. Moving forward, we feel it is essential to continue fostering translingual and transdisciplinary commitments, recognizing the interconnectedness of literature and the potential for lending our senses to worlds and bodies as they work through the health landscapes that run through them.

## WORKS CITED

Fanon, Franz. *Black Skin, White Masks*. Grove Press, 2008.

Nelson, Maggie. *The Art of Cruelty: A Reckoning*. W.W. Norton & Company, 2011.

# Contributors

**Aude Bandini**, PhD, is an associate professor in the Department of Philosophy at Université de Montréal. Her research focuses on social epistemology and the philosophy of medicine. She investigates the nature of experiential knowledge and lay expertise among patients living with chronic illnesses, such as type 1 diabetes. She has also published on epistemic irrationality, with particular attention to phenomena like wilful ignorance and self-deception. Her recent research includes a project examining medical diagnosis as both a speech act and an inquiry process. She currently serves as the director of GRIN (Groupe de Recherche Interuniversitaire sur la Normativité), a prominent research group in philosophy that explores the multifaceted dimensions of affective, social, and epistemic normativity. Additionally, she is the president of the Canadian Society for Epistemology. Dr. Bandini is also an active collaborator in the BETTER project (https://www.type1better.com), a patient-centred initiative co-developed by patient partners, researchers, healthcare providers, and policymakers. The project aims to deepen understanding of the lived experiences of individuals with type 1 diabetes, support advocacy efforts, and promote equitable access to optimal diabetes care across Canada.

**Maxime Raymond Bock**, PhD, was born in Montreal, Quebec, Canada, in 1981. He has published five books of fiction, of which three, *Atavismes* (*Atavisms*, Dalkey Archive, 2015), *Des lames de pierre* (*Baloney*, Coach House, 2016), and *Morel* (QC/Fiction, 2024) have been translated into English. He completed a postdoctoral fellowship at the University of Alberta in 2022 on the problematic and unethical relationship of historical figures Dr. William Beaumont and Alexis Saint-Martin, the *coureur des bois* guinea pig who helped Beaumont ascertain the chemical process of digestion in the 1820s and 1830s.

**Benjamin Gagnon Chainey**, PhD, is a postdoctoral researcher in literature at Université Laval, author, and physiotherapist. In 2022, he completed a PhD in French-language literature, jointly at the Université de Montréal and Nottingham Trent University, on queer aesthetics and phenomenology in late nineteenth-century syphilis and late-twentieth-century AIDS literature, comparing the works of Joris-Karl Huysmans and Hervé Guibert. Since 2023, he has been the communications officer of the Canadian Association for Health Humanities (CAHH). His research and creative texts have appeared in the journals *MuseMedusa*, *Fixxion*, *Interférences littéraires*, *Mœbius*, *SYNAPSIS*, *Lettres françaises*, *Corps*, and *Spirale*, as well as in several edited books. His first novel, *Candy*, was published in September 2022 by Éditions Héliotrope.

**Jonathan Garfinkel**, PhD, is an internationally acclaimed author of six books translated into a dozen languages. He wrote the 2011 Governor General's finalist for drama, *House of Many Tongues*; the memoir *Ambivalence: Crossing the Israel/Palestine Divide* (2008); and the novel *In a Land Without Dogs the Cats Learn to Bark* (2023), in addition to other books of poetry and plays. A frequent contributor to the *Globe and Mail* and *Walrus Magazine*, he was named by the *Toronto Star* as "one to watch." Currently, Jonathan is finishing a research-creation PhD in the field of medical and health humanities in the Department of MLCS at the University of Alberta, a creative non-fiction memoir about living with type one diabetes and Loop. Born in Toronto, raised in Montreal, he lives in Berlin.

**Sander L. Gilman**, PhD, is a distinguished professor emeritus of the liberal arts and sciences as well as emeritus professor of psychiatry at Emory University. A cultural and literary historian, he is the author or editor of over one hundred books. His *"Gebannt in diesem magischen Judenkreis": Essays* appeared with Wallstein Verlag in 2022; his most recent edited volume is *Readers for Life: How Reading and Listening in Childhood Shape Us* (2024). He is the author of the basic study of the visual stereotyping of the mentally ill, *Seeing the Insane*, published by John Wiley and Sons in 1982 (reprinted: 1996 and 2014) as well as the standard study of *Jewish Self-Hatred*, the title of his Johns Hopkins University Press monograph of 1986, which remains in print. He has been a visiting professor at numerous universities in North America, South Africa, the United Kingdom, Germany, Israel, China, and New Zealand. He was president of the Modern Language Association in 1995. He has been awarded a doctor of laws (*honoris causa*) at the University of

Toronto in 1997, elected an honorary professor at the Free University in Berlin (2000), an honorary member of the American Psychoanalytic Association (2007), and made a Fellow of the American Academy of Arts and Sciences (2016).

**Darian Goldin Stahl**, PhD, is an interdisciplinary printmaker whose work explores themes of healthcare, disability, and well-being. After earning an MFA in printmaking from the University of Alberta, she completed a research-creation PhD in humanities at Concordia University, supported by a prestigious Social Sciences and Humanities Research Council of Canada (SSHRC) Vanier scholarship. Her dissertation, *Embodied Books: Experiencing the Health Humanities through Artists' Books*, was published by Peter Lang International Academic Publishers in 2024. Dr. Stahl's novel research was awarded with a SSHRC Banting Postdoctoral Fellowship, which she used to launch the Embodied Books Project at the UNBC Northern Medical Program and Health Arts Research Centre. This initiative empowers intrepid bookmakers to create new artists' books on personal medical experiences. Documentation of this project is available at https://www.embodiedbooks.com. Dr. Stahl's artists' books are included in permanent collections around the world, such as the Wellcome Collection in London, the Moody Library at Baylor University in Texas, and the Thomas Fisher Rare Book Library at the University of Toronto. Her original prints are on permanent display in medical spaces, including the Toronto General Hospital Medical Library and the BARLO Multiple Sclerosis Centre in Toronto. More of her work can be viewed at https://www.dariangoldinstahl.com.

**Eric Jorgensen**, PhD, completed his PhD in the Department of Theater and Dance at the University of California, Santa Barbara with his dissertation *Reacquired: I, Thou, and the American AIDS Play*. The project is a confluence of his work as a professional actor, a performance scholar, and an aid worker. He spent nine years as finance officer with Médecins Sans Frontières/Doctors Without Borders USA including field work in Nigeria, South Sudan, Kenya, Sri Lanka, Uzbekistan, and Jordan. Dr. Jorgensen taught in the Department of Theatre Arts at the University of Wisconsin-La Crosse and served as deputy director of finance at Steppenwolf Theatre Company in Chicago. He is currently visiting assistant professor in the Department of Theatre and Dance at the University of Wyoming.

**Chang-Hee Kim**, PhD, earned his PhD in Literature from the University of Minnesota, Twin Cities, in 2009. He is a professor of English at Yonsei

University in Wonju, South Korea, and served as a Fulbright Mid-Career Research Scholar at the University of California, Irvine, from 2019 to 2020. His current research focuses on critical discourses such as techno-orientalism, artificial intelligence, posthuman studies, and new materialism. Adopting interdisciplinary approaches, he examines Asian American literature and science fiction through the lenses of race, gender, sexuality, and the Anthropocene. Dr. Kim's recent publications include "Parasitic yet Affective Posthumanity in Kogonada's After Yang" (2024), "Posthuman Love for Symbiosis and Coexistence" (2024), "The Virtual Politics of Un-doing Humanity in Speculative Realism: A New Materialist Reading of The Bluest Eye, 'The Birth-Mark,' and *After Yang* " (2023), and "Neoliberal Fantasy and Neocolonial Nightmare in Bong Joon-Ho's Parasite" (2023).

**Eftihia Mihelakis**, PhD, is associate professor of French and Francophone Studies at Brandon University (Manitoba, Canada). She received her PhD in literature with a specialization in literary and intermedial studies from Université de Montréal in 2016. Dr. Mihelakis's fields of interest include twentieth- and twenty-first-century French, francophone, and translingual literatures, feminist theory, health humanities, diasporic writings, and research-creation. Her current Social Sciences and Humanities Research Council of Canada-funded project, *Les écritures de la dépression en contexte de marginalisations*, focuses on the embodiment of depression narratives in desertified spaces. She is the author of *La Virginité en question ou les jeunes filles sans âge* (Presses de l'Université de Montréal, 2017) and co-editor of *Poétiques de l'absence chez Marguerite Duras* (Presses de l'Université du Québec, 2012). Her books have been reviewed in journals such as *Women in French*, *Spirale*, *Voix et Images*, and *Dalhousie French Studies*. She has received multiple awards, including the Scholarly Book Awards | Prix d'aide à l'édition savante (2017 and 2025). Her articles have appeared in *Romanica Cracoviensia, Captures, Tangence*, and *Contemporary French and Francophone Studies*. Her first book of poetry, *Οὔτις Nobody Personne*, will appear in 2026 (Les Herbes rouges).

**Hilary Offman,** MD FRCPC, is a psychiatrist and psychoanalyst with a private practice in Toronto, Canada. She is a lecturer and supervisor in the Department of Psychiatry at the University of Toronto. She is also a supervising analyst, faculty and Board member for the Toronto Institute for Contemporary Psychoanalysis (TICP). She is the former co-chair of the Candidates Committee for the International Association of Relational Psychotherapy and Psychoanalysis (IARPP) and a current member of the IARRP Board of Directors, where she chairs the International Chapters Committee. Her writing interests include themes of otherness, queerness, and fatness. Her papers are used to teach about working psychoanalytically with patients who identify as nonbinary. Her article "Fatphobia Is Real" won the Council for Advancement and Support of Education in Medicine (CASE) Gold Writing Award. Her recent publications include "The Intersectionality of Misogyny: On Being Fat, Female, and Trans," "Under the Gun of Countertransference" in *Psychoanalytic Perspectives* (both 2025 in press), and "Why? July" in the *Annals of Internal Medicine* (2025 in press).

**Fernanda Pérez-Gay Juárez**, PhD, is a medical doctor currently completing a residency in psychiatry. With a PhD in cognitive neuroscience and postdoctoral training in philosophy, she is interested in the intersections between neuroscience, the arts, and the humanities. This interdisciplinary focus shapes her work in health humanities, where she aims to explore innovative ways to integrate scientific and humanistic perspectives to enhance patient care and empathy. Fernanda Pérez Gay Juárez's research spans neural correlates of cognition, use of first-person narratives to foster empathy, and the psychology of conspiracy theories, employing both quantitative and qualitative methods. As a lecturer at McGill University, she has taught neuroscience and cognitive science courses, bringing a nuanced approach to understanding the brain, mind, and human experience. Beyond academia, Fernanda Pérez Gay Juárez is an advocate for mental health awareness and harm-reduction education, communicating insights through public speaking, journalism, and outreach in English, French, and Spanish. Her work's commitment is to bridging the gap between the sciences and humanities to advance healthcare and education.

**Lucille Toth**, PhD, holds a PhD in French and Francophone Studies from the University of Southern California, and specializes in the intersections of dance, migration, and embodiment within the health humanities. She has authored *Danses et pandémies: Du SIDA à la COVID-19* (Nota Bene, 2022) and co-edited *Danse contemporaine et littérature: Entre fictions et performances écrites* (Centre National de la Danse, 2015). Dr. Toth is the recipient of several prestigious awards, including the Early-Career Faculty Excellence Award at the Ohio State University. Her work was also selected for the 2023 Grand Prix du Livre de Montréal, and she was nominated for the 2024 Artists Elevated Award by the Greater Columbus Arts Council. She is the creator of *On Board(hers)*, a dance project for immigrants, where she has led over 50 workshops involving more than 200 participants. Her projects have garnered attention from non-academic outlets, including features in major networks such as NPR (United States), *Le Monde* (France) and *Le Devoir* (Québec).

**Louise Toutée**, MD, PhD, graduated from McGill University with a BA&Sc in cognitive science. Her dissertation looked at the impact of fiction reading on social categorization in theory of mind tasks. She obtained a master's degree in cognitive and evolutionary anthropology from Oxford University and worked as a research associate at the Human Relations Area Files at Yale University, where she studied the cultural adaptations of small-scales societies to climate stresses and shocks. She now works as a science journalist for various Canadian media.

**Julie C. Van Dam**, PhD, is professor of French and gender and sexuality studies (teaching), at the University of Southern California (PhD, UCLA) where she serves as director of undergraduate studies. She is the author of the monograph *Critical Conditions: Illness and Disability in Francophone African and Caribbean Women's Writing* (Lexington, 2012), as well as book chapters and articles in publications such as *Wagadu: Journal of Transnational Women's and Gender Studies, Journal of Literary and Cultural Disability Studies*, and *The Handbook of Postcolonial Disability Studies* (Routledge, 2024). Her most recent project is focused on decolonial approaches to health and crip care in Senegalese urban arts. She teaches on race, gender, disability, health, sexuality, and the history of medicine in postcolonial spaces.

# Index